# ANCIENT HERBAL APOTHECARY:

## Timeless Remedies, Recipes & Secrets for Modern Healing

Sofia Visconti

# FREE GIFT

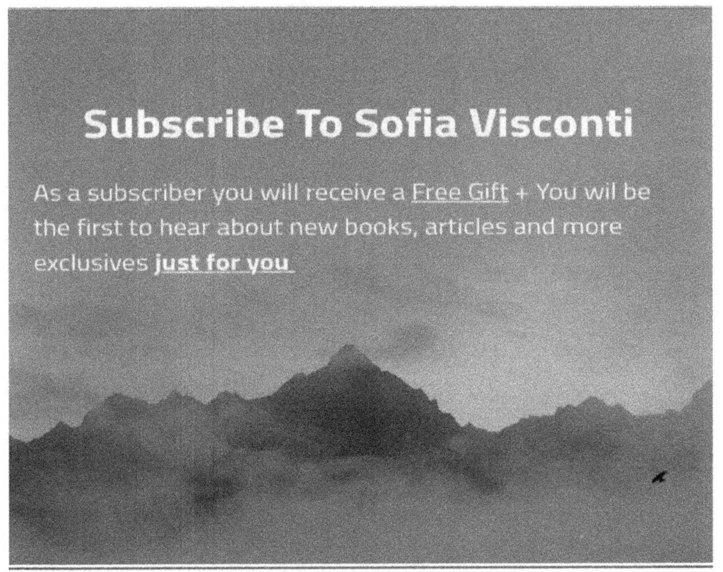


CLICK HERE

Or Visit Below:

https://www.subscribepage.com/svmyth

Simply scan the QR code to join.

# TABLE OF CONTENTS

# Introduction

Imagine a world where the secret to modern health challenges lies not in synthetic drugs but in the time-tested wisdom of herbal medicine. Ancient healers like Hippocrates used natural remedies derived from plants, roots, and herbs—practices that formed the cornerstone of early medicine. Today, blending these age-old techniques with modern science offers a holistic approach to well-being.

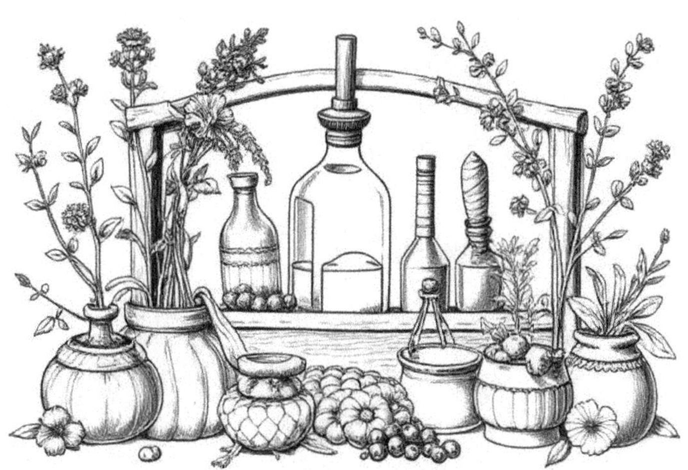

Rather than immediately reaching for a pill, you might soothe a headache with chamomile tea or ease anxiety with the gentle aroma of lavender oil. Herbal medicine isn't just about treating symptoms; it's about creating a balanced lifestyle that includes nutrition, mindfulness, and a deeper connection to nature. In an era marked by rising healthcare costs and environmental concerns, these natural remedies provide accessible, cost-effective alternatives that can complement modern treatments.

Moreover, the resurgence of herbal practices is nurturing community bonds—whether through sharing gardening tips at farmer's markets or exchanging homemade tinctures. This revival reconnects us with traditions that honor the earth and emphasizes our collective responsibility to preserve natural ecosystems.

Begin your journey into the verdant world of herbal medicine, where each plant holds a story of healing, and every natural remedy bridges ancient wisdom and contemporary needs. This exploration invites you to rediscover a path to health that is both timeless and attuned to today's world.

# Chapter 1: The Ancient Roots of Herbal Medicine

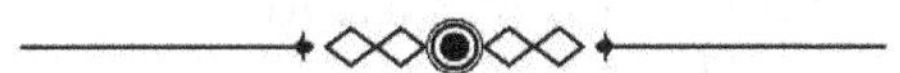

Tracing the history of herbal medicine is like beginning a fascinating journey through time, revealing how ancient civilizations harnessed nature's bounty for healing. From the mystic practices of early societies to the more structured approaches that followed, herbal medicine has always occupied a central place in human culture. These primitive roots have evolved over centuries, influenced by diverse regions and cultures, each contributing unique insights and practices.

The power and allure of herbal remedies lie in their ability to intertwine health and spirituality, creating a tapestry where natural remedies meet cultural beliefs. With each civilization bringing its distinct perspective, the evolution of herbal medicine tells a rich story of innovation, adaptation, and continuity.

In this chapter, we'll explore the foundational history of herbal medicine spanning some of the world's most influential ancient civilizations. We'll uncover why these early societies viewed herbs not just as simple remedies but as essential components of their healthcare systems and spiritual practices.

Through an exploration of the intricacies of Egyptian, Greek, Mesopotamian, and other ancient cultures, we'll see how religious beliefs, societal structures, and daily life were interwoven with botanical knowledge. As we navigate through their contributions, philosophies, and techniques, you'll gain insights into how ancient wisdom laid the groundwork for contemporary herbal practices.

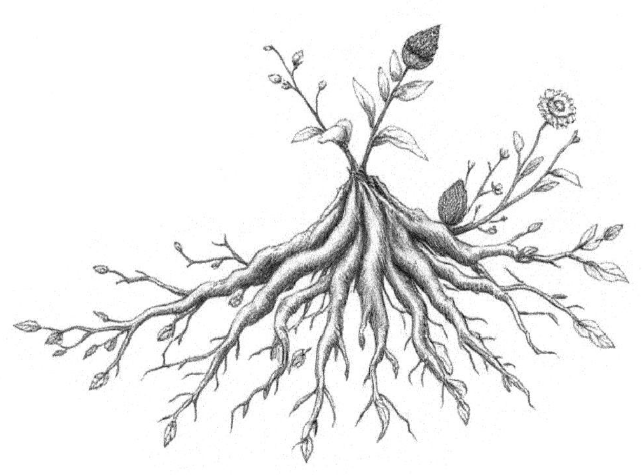

Together, let's unravel the profound impact of these early methods, appreciating how they set the stage for modern understandings of herbal medicine.

## Herbalism in Ancient Egyptian Culture

Herbal medicine was deeply embedded in the fabric of ancient Egyptian societies, playing a crucial role in combining health, spirituality, and daily life. For starters, skilled herbalists held a prestigious position, often serving the elite. These practitioners were not only medical figures but also spiritual guides, as their knowledge of herbs was believed to connect the physical and spiritual realms. Their ability to cure ailments and create herbal potions was seen as almost magical, elevating their status within the social hierarchy.

In addition to medicinal uses, herbs were an essential component of mummification, a practice fundamental to the Egyptian afterlife beliefs. The Egyptians believed that preserving the body with herbs ensured a successful journey to the afterlife and eternal life thereafter. Various aromatic plants and resins, such as myrrh and frankincense, were meticulously applied during the mummification process. This use of herbs highlights their dual role in both sustaining life and ensuring a sacred transition through death.

The sophistication of Egyptian herbalism is further exemplified by the existence of extensive papyrus scrolls dedicated to botanical knowledge. Manuscripts like the Ebers Papyrus serve as testaments to the Egyptians' advanced understanding of plants and their properties. These documents reveal a systematic approach to herbal knowledge, listing remedies for various ailments and illustrating the practical application of herbs in everyday life. The detailed records emphasize an intention to preserve knowledge for future generations, showcasing a profound respect for documentation and learning.

Moreover, certain herbs held divine associations, intimately linking them with religious practices and rituals.

For instance, sacred plants like the lotus were not only used for their therapeutic benefits but also incorporated into ceremonies designed to harmonize health and spirituality. Such rituals aimed to balance an individual's physical health and spiritual well-being, reflecting the broader Egyptian worldview where medicine and magic were inseparable.

The cultural symbolism of these herbs cannot be overstated. Beyond their practical applications, plants like papyrus became symbols of life and growth and were frequently represented in art and architecture. The reverence for these plants illustrates their importance beyond mere physical healing; they played a vital role in expressing the Egyptians' connection with the divine and the natural world.

## Greek Contributions to Herbal Knowledge

Ancient Greek thinkers laid some of the foundational stones in the development of herbal medicine, offering insights that have percolated through centuries to inform modern practices.

Central to this legacy is the Hippocratic Corpus, a collection of texts attributed to or inspired by Hippocrates, a figure often hailed as the father of medicine. Unlike mystical approaches that dominated earlier thought, these writings emphasized observation and rational analysis of the human body in health and illness. Within this framework, herbs played a crucial role; they were viewed not merely as ingredients with magical properties but as tools for restoring balance within the body.

The humoral theory, which proposed that health depended on balancing bodily fluids called humors, tied directly into herbal prescriptions and treatments. This rational approach influenced generations of medical practitioners, shaping Western medicine's trajectory away from superstition toward empirical methods (*Ancient Greek Medicine*, 2008).

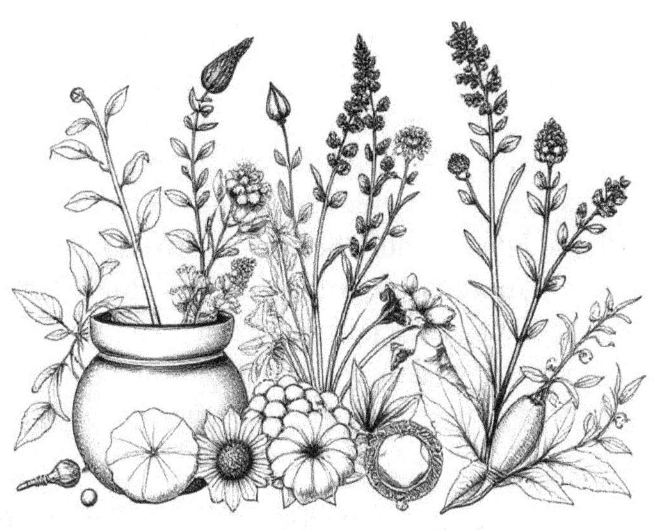

Another critical aspect of ancient Greek contributions was their systematic cataloging of plants. The Greeks were among the first to document various plant species meticulously, linking them to their therapeutic uses. These lists represented an early scientific attempt to understand and connect nature with health. They did not simply list plants but described their effects and potential applications, effectively laying the groundwork for pharmacology. Such documentation paved the way for subsequent generations to explore, experiment, and expand upon this foundation, allowing for a more structured understanding of how plants could be harnessed for medicinal purposes.

The work of Theophrastus, a student of Aristotle, further advanced this botanical exploration. Often considered the father of botany, Theophrastus undertook extensive studies and classifications of plants, contributing significantly to the knowledge base essential for herbal medicine. His inquiries into plant structure, reproduction, and growth patterns provided a deeper insight into the natural world. By organizing plants into different categories based on characteristics, he offered a system that allowed for easier identification and application of herbs in medical contexts (Totelin, 2014). This classification was crucial because it marked an evolution from viewing plants as mysterious entities to understanding them as part of a broader ecological and biological system.

Greek literature also provides rich references to herbs, highlighting their societal roles and enhancing our understanding of ancient worldviews. In epic tales and myths, herbs are often depicted as powerful agents that heroes and gods wield. For example, in Homer's epics, certain plants are endowed with divine attributes, capable of healing wounds or inducing transformations. Such narratives showcase the high regard in which these cultures held herbal knowledge and its integration into everyday life and spirituality.

These literary depictions served multiple purposes: they chronicled herbal use, transmitted cultural values, and reflected the collective consciousness of the interplay between humans and nature. By weaving herbs into stories, the Greeks communicated both practical information and philosophical reflections on health, illness, and the environment. This dual function of storytelling helped preserve herbal knowledge across generations, embedding it within the fabric of cultural identity and practice.

Furthermore, it's important to consider how the Greeks' understanding of herbs spread beyond their own borders, influencing other civilizations through trade and interaction. As Greek cultures intersected with those of Egypt, Persia, and Rome, their herbal practices and philosophies disseminated widely. Such exchanges enriched the diversity of medicinal approaches in antiquity, creating a dynamic fusion that bolstered the overall knowledge pool available to ancient societies.

The thoughtful contributions of Greek thinkers declare the importance of approaching herbal medicine as an empirical science rather than a mysterious art. Their emphasis on observation, classification, and documentation established methodologies that continue to resonate in contemporary herbal and medical practices. In many ways, the social and scientific advancements made by these early pioneers set the stage for the eventual emergence of more sophisticated pharmacological studies and holistic health practices.

## Mesopotamian Herbal Texts

The history of herbal medicine is as rich as it is ancient, and nowhere is this more evident than in Mesopotamia. This cradle of civilization provides some of the earliest documentation of organized medicinal practices through its extensive collection of cuneiform tablets. In these tablets, we see the beginnings of a structured approach to herbal medicine that would influence cultures for millennia to come.

The Mesopotamian people meticulously recorded their medical knowledge on hundreds of thousands of these clay tablets, with some dating back to the mid-fourth millennium BC (Boeck, 2020). Due to the durability of these baked clay records, modern historians and archaeologists have gained invaluable insights into the pharmacological acumen of our ancestors.

These texts reveal that the Mesopotamians had developed a sophisticated understanding of herbal pharmacology, using detailed prescriptions and treatments—often involving multiple formulations for a single ailment. The systematic use of herbs was not just ad-hoc; it reflected an advanced approach to medicine that laid the groundwork for future medical traditions globally.

Religious figures often played a central role in the management of herbal knowledge within Mesopotamia.

Shamans and priests were the custodians of this critical information, which created a blend of spiritualism and early medical science in practice. The intertwining roles of religion and medicine manifested in rituals and incantations believed to aid healing processes.

For instance, divination techniques such as extispicy—not unlike reading tea leaves today—were employed to diagnose illnesses and prescribe cures (Boeck, 2020). This combination of spirituality with practical healthcare highlights the holistic view the Mesopotamians held toward health and disease—a perspective still valued in alternative medicine practices today.

One of the most compelling aspects of Mesopotamian herbal texts is their documentation of practical remedies. These records include not only lists of plants and their uses but also elaborate descriptions of how to identify, harvest, and prepare medicinal ingredients effectively. Key reference works like the Uruanna: maštakal lexicon cataloged around 1,300 drug terms, covering approximately 340 plant species and indicating an encyclopedic effort to document the natural world's medicinal offerings (Boeck, 2020).

Mesopotamian healers exhibited remarkable competence, with prescriptions that addressed symptoms comparable to those found in modern medicine. Their methodologies reflect a foundational approach to healthcare that stresses observation, trial, and documentation—a precursor to empirical scientific methods.

Cultural interactions across the ancient world facilitated the exchange of herbal knowledge, illustrating an interconnected landscape of traditional medicine. Mesopotamia, being strategically located amidst several civilizations such as the Egyptian, Persian, and Greek, became a conduit for sharing medicinal practices (Boeck, 2020). Trade routes not only carried goods but also allowed for the transmission of ideas, leading to enriched medicinal knowledge pools.

For example, records from King Assurbanipal's library—the largest surviving collection of medical texts—showcase a plethora of entries that contain contributions from various neighboring cultures, thus highlighting the dynamic nature of knowledge diffusion (Norman, 2014).

Moreover, the enduring influence of these Mesopotamian texts underscores their importance in shaping the course of herbal medicine. Modern botanists and pharmacologists can trace certain herbal preparations and theories back to these early manuscripts. Despite the challenges of language translation and the fragmented state of some texts, the underlying principles have been passed down through generations, offering a testament to the robustness of Mesopotamian wisdom.

## Cultural Symbolism and Exchange of Herbal Practices

Herbal medicine has deep roots stretching across various ancient civilizations, where it was more than a mere practice for healing. It held symbolic significance linked to deities, thereby enhancing its societal prestige. In numerous cultures, herbs weren't just medicinal; they were often seen as gifts from the gods or embodiments of divine will.

For instance, in ancient Egypt, herbs such as basil and thyme were associated with specific deities, elevating their importance beyond their physical healing properties. Similarly, in India, the revered plant Tulsi was considered sacred to Hindu gods, highlighting the revered status of certain herbs (Elendu, 2024). This connection between herbs and spirituality reinforced their value and cemented their presence within cultural practices.

Ritual uses of herbs underscored their role in bridging health and sacred practices. Many civilizations employed herbs in religious ceremonies and rituals aimed at promoting both physical and spiritual well-being. The burning of sage in Native American rituals serves as a prime example of how herbs bridged the gap between tangible health benefits and spiritual purification.

Ancient Greeks also used a variety of herbs in religious offerings, believing in their power to purify and protect against evil (*A Guide to Traditional Herbalism Across Cultures*, 2024). Such ritual use of herbs illustrates their dual function in serving the body while feeding the spirit, thus blending the lines between health and faith.

Exchanges of herbal knowledge between societies depict the dynamic diffusion of medicinal practices, further illustrating how interconnected early civilizations were due to trade and travel. As merchants and travelers moved along routes like the Silk Road, they carried not only goods but also valuable herbal knowledge. This sharing of information led to a fusion of different traditions and an enrichment of local practices.

For example, the introduction of Chinese herbal remedies into Persia and later into Europe demonstrates this cultural exchange (Elendu, 2024). These interactions enabled societies to adapt and enhance their own medicinal practices by incorporating insights from other cultures.

The fusion of herbal traditions across cultures enriched the complexity and diversity of ancient healing methods. When we examine the traditional practices of a civilization like China, for instance, it's clear that their use of herbs was an amalgamation of indigenous methods, combined with influences from neighboring regions.

Similar patterns of integration can be observed in Ayurvedic practices in India, which meld local traditions with insights gained from interactions with Greek and Persian traders (*A Guide to Traditional Herbalism Across Cultures*, 2024). This cross-pollination of ideas contributed to a richer, more complex tapestry of herbal knowledge that could address a wider range of ailments and conditions.

Cultural exchange was also pivotal in advancing the scientific understanding of herbal medicine. In ancient Greece, scholars like Hippocrates and, later, Galen were heavily influenced by Egyptian and Mesopotamian knowledge. Their systematic study of plants laid foundational principles for what would become Western medicine (Elendu, 2024). The intersection of different herbal traditions prompted an evolution in thought processes, moving from mystical interpretations toward more empirical observations and categorizations of herb-derived treatments.

The synthesis of diverse herbal practices gave rise to innovative treatments and techniques. For instance, Mediterranean herbs such as rosemary and oregano found their way into Middle Eastern pharmacology, where they were studied for new therapeutic applications. Conversely, Eastern spices and herbs made their mark on European cuisine, sparking culinary revolutions that also enhanced health. This back-and-forth exchange catalyzed a global appreciation and utilization of herbs which persists today in countless complementary medicinal practices worldwide.

Moreover, the mutual respect and learning that stemmed from these exchanges fostered a sense of unity and shared purpose among different cultures. By valuing each other's contributions, these ancient societies promoted a collaborative atmosphere that encouraged an ongoing exploration and understanding of the natural world. Such partnerships exemplified the idea of using collective wisdom to tackle common challenges, especially regarding health and wellness (Elendu, 2024).

## Bringing It All Together

Throughout this chapter, we've journeyed through the fascinating history of herbal medicine across ancient civilizations. From the mystical uses of herbs in ancient Egypt that intertwined health and spirituality to the methodical cataloging by Greek thinkers, which laid the groundwork for modern practices, it's clear just how integral these natural wonders were in shaping cultural approaches to health. We looked into the treasures of Mesopotamian texts, where, even then, medicine was emerging as a blend of practical knowledge and spiritualism. Altogether, they reveal a world where plants were not just medicinal tools but also symbols deeply embedded in society's way of life.

What stands out is the interconnectedness of ancient societies through trade and knowledge exchange, enriching each other's understanding of herbal medicine. This cultural fusion allowed for a diverse and dynamic knowledge pool, laying strong foundations for future generations. Whether it was the sacred plant rituals or the empirical observations that aided in the transition from mysticism to science, the imprint of these early pioneers is undeniable. Looking back at how different cultures revered and utilized plants can inspire us today to appreciate and explore the wealth of natural solutions we have at our disposal.

# Chapter 2: Nature's Pharmacy–Key Plants and Their Ancient Uses

Discovering the secrets behind nature's pharmacy can open a world of fascinating insights about the plants we often overlook. For centuries, many cultures have relied on natural remedies to heal and sustain health. Plants are not just for food or decoration; they have played a crucial role in medicine across various civilizations. From easing painful ailments with willow bark to harnessing the antimicrobial powers of garlic, ancient people used the earth's flora in resourceful ways that now form the bedrock of our modern understanding of plant-based therapies.

This chapter will explore some of the key plants historically utilized by the early pioneers of medicine. We'll examine the use of willow bark as a natural painkiller, revered long before any synthetic alternatives existed, and garlic's legacy as a powerful antibiotic alongside modern validations of its efficacy. Furthermore, we will explore the multifaceted benefits of ginseng, esteemed for its ability to enhance stamina and mental sharpness over the ages.

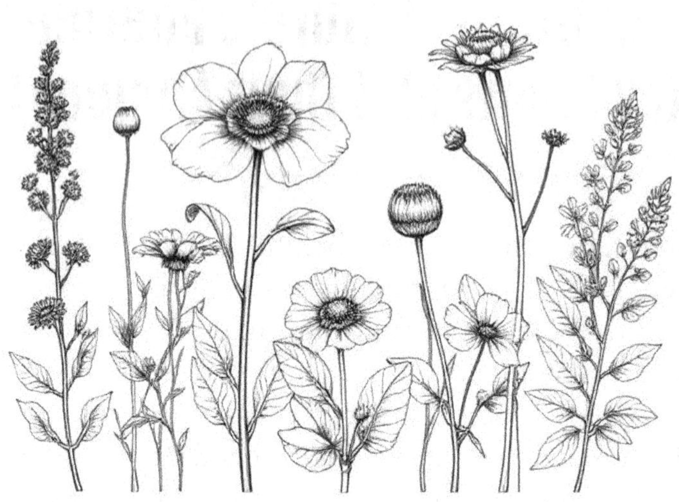

Through this lens, you'll appreciate how age-old practices inform our current medicinal approaches, blending tradition with innovation to enrich contemporary healthcare. Whether you're considering these plants for personal wellness or simply curious about their history, there's plenty to learn and rediscover from the past.

## Willow Bark: The Ancient Pain Reliever

Throughout history, willow bark has been a cornerstone in herbal medicine for alleviating pain. Ancient civilizations recognized its potential as a natural remedy. For instance, the Greeks and Egyptians utilized it for treating headaches and joint pain, cases that likely included early notions of arthritis. Hippocrates, the father of modern medicine, even referred to chewing on willow leaves to reduce fever and inflammation as far back as 400

BC (Icahn School of Medicine at Mount Sinai, n.d.). This historical tradition highlights willow bark's long-standing role in managing painful conditions, underscoring the wisdom of our ancestors.

The key to understanding willow bark's efficacy lies in its active ingredient, salicin. Salicin is a chemical compound that plays a significant role in pain relief. When ingested, salicin is converted into salicylic acid in the body, which then works to reduce pain and inflammation much like aspirin. In fact, scientists in the 19th century used salicin as the basis for developing modern aspirin.

The slow release of salicylic acid from willow bark means that its effects are gradual but can be longer-lasting compared to direct aspirin consumption (Icahn School of Medicine at Mount Sinai, n.d.). This process provides a fascinating insight into how ancient remedies have informed and shaped contemporary medicines, effectively bridging past knowledge with present-day science.

For those interested in integrating willow bark into their wellness routine, it's quite possible to craft homemade teas and tinctures. These methods of preparation ensure users can benefit from the bark's medicinal properties while controlling the dosage.

To make a willow bark tea, you would typically steep one to two teaspoons of dried willow bark in boiling water for about ten minutes. Once strained, this concoction can be sipped slowly (Lin et al., 2023). Similarly, tinctures involve soaking willow bark in alcohol for several weeks, allowing the beneficial compounds to infuse the liquid fully. Such preparations not only make it accessible for personal use but also empower individuals to take an active role in their health management.

Despite its benefits, it is crucial to approach willow bark with informed caution. Consulting healthcare professionals before incorporating it into your regimen is wise, especially if you're currently on medications. Willow bark contains salicylates similar to aspirin, which can lead to adverse effects when mixed with certain drugs or in people with specific medical conditions such as asthma or gastrointestinal issues (Icahn School of Medicine at Mount Sinai, n.d.). Notably, it is advised against use during pregnancy or breastfeeding due to potential risks to both mother and child.

Moreover, while its side effects tend to be mild, some individuals may experience stomach upset or allergic reactions. Understanding these risks reinforces the importance of professional guidance and adherence to recommended doses. Overconsumption can cause more severe symptoms like nausea or skin rashes, emphasizing the necessity for prudent usage.

## Garlic: Nature's Antibiotic

Garlic, a staple in kitchens around the world, has played an integral role in traditional medicine for centuries. Its antibacterial properties were highly valued by ancient civilizations, notably the Egyptians, who used it to support the health of laborers building monumental structures like the pyramids. This usage underscores its historical importance, as garlic was believed to help maintain the workers' strength and resilience against potential infections as they worked.

The magic behind garlic's efficacy lies in allicin, a compound that forms when garlic cloves are crushed or chopped. Allicin's potent antimicrobial effects have been well-documented, with modern scientific studies confirming garlic's ability to combat various pathogens, including multi-drug-resistant strains (Bhatwalkar et al., 2021). This makes garlic a formidable weapon against bacteria. Research highlights the chemical reactions of allicin with thiol groups in enzymes, which involves disrupting essential bacterial processes and rendering them ineffective (Ankri & Mirelman, 1999).

Incorporating garlic into daily life offers an easy and natural way to boost health. Garlic-infused oils or teas serve as practical remedies, tapping into both its flavor and therapeutic potential. These preparations can be simple to make at home and provide an opportunity to harness garlic's benefits regularly. For those interested in exploring this path, you can prepare garlic oil by gently heating crushed garlic in olive oil to release its active compounds and then straining it for use in cooking or as a topical application.

However, while adding garlic to one's routine can be advantageous, it's important to remain mindful of possible side effects. Raw garlic is known to cause gastrointestinal discomfort, including bloating and gas, in some people. Furthermore, garlic may interact with certain medications, including anticoagulants, which can increase the risk of bleeding, particularly before surgical procedures. Thus, a balanced approach to consumption is necessary, emphasizing moderation and, if needed, consultation with a healthcare professional to avoid adverse effects.

## Ginseng: The Adaptogenic Marvel

Ginseng, often heralded as a cornerstone of Chinese medicine, has long held a reputation for enhancing vitality and mental acuity. The efficacy of this revered *panacea* is backed by centuries of use and modern scientific validation. Chinese herbalists have historically championed ginseng for its powerful adaptogenic properties that aid in boosting the body's resilience to stress while bolstering immune function—a dual benefit that enhances overall well-being.

Ginsenosides, the active compounds within ginseng, are critical in driving these benefits. These saponins are noteworthy not only for their complex chemical structure but also for their therapeutic effects. Ginsenosides improve the body's stress response mechanisms and enhance immune system capabilities. Modern studies echo ancient wisdom, showcasing how these compounds interact with the central nervous system to bolster cognitive functions, potentially slowing neurodegenerative processes (Wee et al., 2011). Such findings support the traditional belief in ginseng's role as an agent of longevity and vitality.

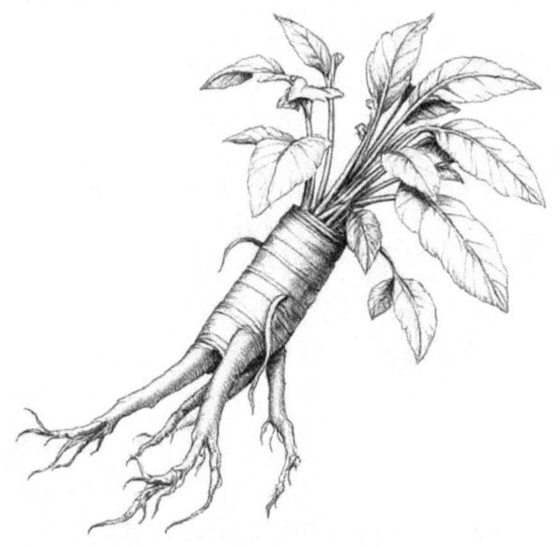

While Chinese herbalists were among the pioneers in harnessing the benefits of ginseng, contemporary practices have adapted these methods to suit modern lifestyles without compromising efficacy. The preparation of ginseng tea and tinctures stands out as a classic example of this blend between old and new. Making ginseng tea is straightforward: slice dried ginseng root into thin pieces, add them to boiling water, and steep for about ten minutes. The resulting brew is a time-honored way to consume ginseng, facilitating mental clarity and energy in a convenient manner that fits today's world.

Additionally, crafting a tincture offers another practical approach. This involves cutting ginseng root and soaking it in a high-proof alcohol like vodka for several weeks.

The alcohol acts as a solvent, extracting valuable compounds from the ginseng, producing a potent liquid form that can be taken in small doses. Both the tea and tincture methods underscore the versatility of ginseng preparations, allowing individuals to tailor intake to their specific health needs and preferences.

However, as demand for ginseng has surged—particularly in North America and Europe, it becomes crucial to verify the quality and sources of ginseng products. Differences in species, cultivation methods, and processing can significantly affect the efficacy of the product. Ensuring that one purchases ginseng from reputable sources helps ensure purity and potency while minimizing the risk of adverse interactions with medications.

Certified suppliers who adhere to sustainable harvesting practices and comply with quality assurance standards are recommended. Additionally, awareness of potential interactions with other herbs or medications is essential, especially since ginseng's stimulating properties might exacerbate conditions like high blood pressure or lead to interactions with anticoagulants. Consulting healthcare professionals before incorporating ginseng into one's regimen ensures safety and maximizes health benefits.

## Practical Guide to Herbal Remedies

If you're looking to harness the power of nature for your wellness goals, integrating plants like willow bark, garlic, and ginseng into your daily routine can be a great start. These ancient remedies have stood the test of time, offering natural solutions that are both effective and easy to prepare at home.

Let's kick off with willow bark. Known for its pain-relieving properties, willow bark is a fantastic alternative for mild discomfort. For pain relief, a common dosage of willow bark is 1–3 grams of dried bark per day, brewed as tea or taken in supplement form. Its active compound, salicin, works similarly to aspirin, helping to reduce headaches, muscle pain, and inflammation.

Alternatively, you can create a tincture by soaking dried bark in alcohol for several weeks, shaking occasionally. Once it's ready, a few drops under the tongue can provide relief. Remember, though, to consult your healthcare provider before use, especially if you're on medication (Jahromi et al., 2021).

Garlic isn't just for adding flavor to your meals; it's also a potent medicinal tool. Incorporating garlic into your diet enhances your immune system and aids in combating infections. Crushing fresh garlic cloves and letting them sit for a few minutes releases allicin, its key active component. You can mix crushed garlic with honey for a sweet and savory remedy or add it to warm olive oil to make an infused oil. Use this oil in cooking or as a salad dressing to reap its health benefits. Just ensure moderation in use to avoid any potential gastrointestinal disturbances (*Willow Is a Valuable Medicine for Rheumatic Conditions*, 2025).

Ginseng, revered in traditional Chinese medicine, is perfect for boosting vitality. Ginseng is usually taken in doses of 200–400 mg of extract per day or 1–2 grams of dried root brewed as tea. Known for boosting energy, improving focus, and supporting the immune system, ginseng is a powerful adaptogen that helps the body manage stress. In addition, ginsenoside compounds support immunity and stress resistance. Balancing these traditional approaches with modern convenience makes ginseng accessible to everyone, whether you're brewing tea on a chilly morning or using a tincture during a busy day.

Safety should be at the forefront of any herbal regimen. While these plants offer many benefits, it's crucial to respect their potency. Always source high-quality ingredients from reputable suppliers to ensure purity and avoid contaminants. Be aware of potential interactions between herbs and medications or pre-existing conditions. Consulting with a healthcare professional can provide certainty when trying new herbal remedies.

## Herbal Remedies: Practical Applications of Willow Bark, Garlic, and Ginseng

Having explored the rich history, medicinal properties, and traditional uses of willow bark, garlic, and ginseng, you may now be curious about how to bring these age-old remedies into your everyday routine. The following section offers clear, step-by-step recipes to create your own herbal remedies at home. These practical instructions provide a natural extension of the chapter's narrative—turning historical insights and scientific knowledge into accessible, hands-on wellness practices.

## Willow Bark Remedies

Willow bark has long been celebrated for its natural pain-relieving properties. Below are two simple methods to harness its benefits in your own home.

### Willow Bark Tea

For pain relief, let the ancient power of willow bark tea work its magic, swiftly melting away any discomfort and invigorating you with every soothing sip.

**Ingredients:**

- 1–2 tsp of dried willow bark
- 1 cup of boiling water

**Instructions:**

1. Place the dried willow bark in a teapot or heatproof cup.
2. Pour one cup of boiling water over the bark.
3. Steep for about 10 minutes.
4. Strain the tea into a cup.
5. Sip slowly, allowing the gentle release of salicin to ease discomfort.

**Contraindications:**

- Due to its salicylate content, avoid using it if you are allergic to aspirin, on blood-thinning medication, or have a sensitive stomach.
- Pregnant or breastfeeding women should consult a healthcare professional before use.

## Willow Bark Tincture

Willow bark tincture delivers a concentrated burst of nature's power, quickly easing aches and inflammation with every drop, offering a fast and effective remedy.

**Ingredients:**

- Dried willow bark
- High-proof alcohol (such as vodka)

**Instructions:**

1. Fill a clean jar about halfway with dried willow bark.
2. Pour enough high-proof alcohol over the bark to fully submerge it.
3. Seal the jar tightly and store it in a cool, dark place.
4. Shake the jar gently every day for 3–4 weeks.
5. Strain the infusion through a fine mesh or cheesecloth.
6. Transfer the liquid into a dark glass bottle for storage.

**Contraindications:**

- Not recommended for individuals allergic to salicylates or those taking other anti-inflammatory or blood-thinning medications.
- Pregnant or breastfeeding women should consult a healthcare professional prior to use.

## Garlic Remedies

Garlic's powerful antimicrobial and immune-boosting qualities have been revered since ancient times. The following recipes will show you how to incorporate garlic into your wellness routine in both culinary and therapeutic forms.

### Garlic-Infused Oil

For immune support, let the ancient power of garlic-infused oil work its magic, unleashing potent antimicrobial benefits and invigorating your well-being with every golden drop.

**Ingredients:**

- 3–4 garlic cloves, crushed
- ½ cup olive oil

**Instructions:**

1. Crush the garlic cloves and let them sit for about 5 minutes to activate the allicin.
2. In a small saucepan, combine the crushed garlic with olive oil.

3. Warm the mixture over low heat for 10–15 minutes (do not let it boil to preserve active compounds).
4. Remove from heat and allow the oil to cool.
5. Strain the oil into a clean container.
6. Use this oil in cooking or as a gentle topical antimicrobial application.

**Contraindications:**

- May cause gastrointestinal discomfort in sensitive individuals; use externally with caution if you have sensitive skin.
- Consult a healthcare professional if you are pregnant or taking blood-thinning medications.

### Garlic and Honey Remedy

The soothing power of garlic and honey, combining two age-old natural remedies, can help boost your body's defenses and provide a nourishing, healing touch with every spoonful.

**Ingredients:**

- 2–3 garlic cloves, finely crushed or minced
- 1 tbsp raw honey

**Instructions:**

1. Finely crush or mince the garlic cloves.
2. Mix the garlic with the raw honey in a small bowl.
3. Let the mixture sit for 5–10 minutes to activate the allicin.

4. Consume a small spoonful daily or mix with warm water as desired.

**Contraindications:**

- Start with small amounts to assess tolerance, as raw garlic may cause gastrointestinal discomfort in some individuals.
- Those with garlic allergies should avoid this remedy.
- Pregnant or breastfeeding women should consult a healthcare professional before use.

## Ginseng Remedies

Renowned for its adaptogenic properties and ability to boost vitality, ginseng remains a staple in both ancient and modern herbal practices. Here are two easy recipes to enjoy ginseng's benefits in a form that suits your lifestyle.

### Ginseng Tea

Let the ancient power of ginseng tea awaken your senses and energize your body and mind with every invigorating sip while boosting your resilience and focus.

**Ingredients:**

- 1 small piece (about 1–2 inches) of dried ginseng root, sliced thinly
- 1 cup of boiling water

**Instructions:**

1. Thinly slice the dried ginseng root.

2. Place the slices in a teapot or heatproof cup.
3. Pour boiling water over the ginseng.
4. Allow the tea to steep for approximately 10 minutes.
5. Strain and enjoy while warm.

**Optional:** Enhance flavor with a touch of honey or lemon.

**Contraindications:**

- May interact with medications for diabetes or blood pressure; consult a healthcare professional if you are on such medications.
- Not recommended for pregnant women unless advised by a healthcare provider.

## Ginseng Tincture

Let the ancient power of ginseng tincture work its magic, infusing every drop with concentrated energy and focus to awaken your inner strength.

**Ingredients:**

- Dried or fresh ginseng root, chopped into small pieces
- High-proof alcohol (like vodka)

**Instructions:**

1. Place the chopped ginseng root in a clean jar, filling it about halfway.

2. Pour enough high-proof alcohol over the root to cover it completely.
3. Seal the jar tightly and store it in a cool, dark area.
4. Shake the jar gently every day for 3–4 weeks.
5. Strain the liquid to remove the ginseng pieces.
6. Transfer the tincture into a dark glass bottle for storage.

**Contraindications:**

- May cause insomnia or increased heart rate in sensitive individuals; monitor your body's response.
- Consult a healthcare professional if you are pregnant, breastfeeding, or on prescription medications.

## Safety and Best Practices

Before integrating any herbal remedy into your daily routine, remember these key points:

- **Consultation:** Always consult with a healthcare professional before starting new herbal remedies, particularly if you are on medications or have pre-existing health conditions.
- **Quality:** Source high-quality, organic herbs from reputable suppliers.
- **Moderation:** Begin with small doses to test your body's reaction before increasing intake.

- **Storage:** Store your homemade remedies in dark glass bottles and in a cool, dry place to maintain their potency.

## Bringing It All Together

Exploring the uses of willow bark, garlic, and ginseng and tracing their applications from ancient times to today reveals how deeply rooted they are in traditional medicine. These natural remedies offer benefits ranging from pain relief and antimicrobial properties to enhanced vitality and resilience.

By understanding their active components—like salicin in willow bark, allicin in garlic, and ginsenosides in ginseng, we see how each herb contributes to health and wellness uniquely. What's truly intriguing is how this historical knowledge continues to impact modern-day practices, bridging the gap between ancestral wisdom and contemporary science.

As we consider incorporating these herbs into our lives, it's essential to approach them with a sense of curiosity and caution. While they offer exciting possibilities for enhancing well-being, one must be mindful of their potency and potential interactions with medications or existing health conditions. Sourcing high-quality ingredients, being aware of recommended dosages, and seeking professional advice can help ensure a safe and beneficial herbal journey.

Whether you're sipping on willow bark tea for gentle pain relief, enjoying the immune-boosting powers of garlic, or tapping into ginseng's energizing effects, these age-old remedies continue to enrich our modern lives!

# Chapter 3: The Forgotten Herbalists in Times of Crisis

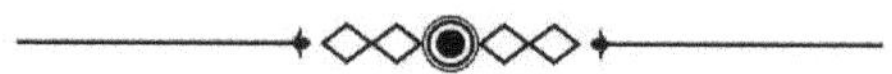

Forgotten herbalists played a pivotal role in times of crisis, wielding the ancient wisdom of herbal remedies when conventional medicine was out of reach. Herbal practices have existed throughout history as an accessible form of healing, offering communities a lifeline during pandemics and other widespread health challenges. Their use highlights humanity's age-old reliance on nature to cope with ailments, serving both physical and emotional needs during tumultuous periods. These natural remedies not only served as practical solutions but also symbolized hope and resilience for those living through dark times.

In this chapter, we'll look into how these herbal solutions were employed during historical crises, focusing specifically on their impact during the Black Plague. We'll explore the unique array of plants that became essential in treating symptoms and preventing disease spread.

Furthermore, this chapter discusses the role of herbalists, who emerged as community heroes, integrating holistic and communal approaches to healthcare. By exploring various herbal concoctions and their applications, you will gain insight into the broader postcrisis societal shifts toward natural medicine. This exploration will reveal the transformative potential of integrating traditional practices with modern medical approaches, highlighting a legacy that continues to influence today's healthcare landscape.

## Herbal Methods During the Black Plague

In times of crisis, herbal remedies have historically been a cornerstone for communities battling widespread disease. During one of history's deadliest pandemics, the reliance on herbs such as yarrow, sage, and chamomile became pivotal. These plants were widely used to combat symptoms like fever and inflammation, showcasing how their essential properties promote healing. Yarrow, for example, was known for its ability to reduce fevers, sage offered antiseptic qualities, and chamomile provided soothing relief for various ailments (Bharathi et al., 2025).

During the pandemic, historical recipes for herbal tinctures were crafted not just for ingestion but also for air purification. This practice underscores an early understanding of preventive measures against disease spread, as communities sought to cleanse their environments to protect against airborne pathogens. Tinctures made from herbs with strong antimicrobial properties served as rudimentary yet effective disinfectants. The use of these tinctures reflects a blend of traditional wisdom and emerging public health needs, emphasizing the community's trust in natural solutions when faced with limited medical resources.

Herbalists emerged as crucial figures in public health during this period. These practitioners often operated at the intersection of medicine and community care, offering both herbal remedies and guidance. Their work highlighted a deep-rooted trust in holistic approaches and alternative healthcare systems. Communities relied heavily on herbalists not only for physical remedies but also for comfort and reassurance amidst the uncertainty of the pandemic. This reliance forged stronger bonds within communities, proving the resilience and adaptability of people utilizing what was accessible to them.

The societal impact of this herbal reliance was significant. As conventional medicine struggled to keep pace with the crisis, there was a tangible shift toward integrating holistic health practices into everyday life. Communities began to favor a more comprehensive approach to health, one that acknowledged the benefits of blending traditional and modern medical practices. This shift revealed an increased postcrisis awareness and acceptance of alternative healthcare methods, leading to a broader integration of natural remedies into mainstream medical care.

Reflecting on the lessons learned from such historical reliance on herbal remedies reveals several key insights. Firstly, it demonstrates the importance of preserving traditional knowledge about medicinal plants. Such knowledge proved invaluable in providing immediate relief and long-term health strategies when conventional resources were scarce. Secondly, it emphasizes the need for preventive measures in managing public health, wherein simple acts like air purification using herbal tinctures can significantly curb disease spread.

A guideline we can derive from examining these historical instances is that preventive measures play a critical role in managing health crises. Proactively engaging in practices that limit disease transmission using available natural resources can be immensely beneficial. This teaches us that incorporating preventive strategies along with treatment can strengthen community resilience against future pandemics.

Moreover, these historical experiences underline the value of trusting and empowering local healthcare providers like herbalists. In times when modern medicine may not immediately reach everyone, local experts become vital in disseminating health information and treatments tailored to the culture and region. Supporting and integrating these practitioners into broader healthcare frameworks ensures a layered and inclusive response to health crises.

Another important lesson from this history is the potential for societal transformation through holistic practices. By embracing a more integrative approach to health, communities not only responded effectively to immediate threats but also laid the groundwork for enhanced well-being and health consciousness. Post the pandemic, many continued to adopt holistic health practices, reflecting a permanent change in lifestyle and community health perspectives.

## Herbal Preparations Used to Treat War Injuries

In times of war and crisis, herbal remedies have often played a crucial role in treating physical trauma. One might not immediately think of herbs when considering medical treatments, but the application of plants like comfrey, calendula, and arnica for wounds is well-documented. These herbs possess remarkable healing and anti-inflammatory properties that make them invaluable in such situations.

Comfrey, known scientifically as *Symphytum officinale*, has been used throughout history for its ability to accelerate the healing process. Traditionally referred to as "knitbone," this herb contains allantoin, which promotes new cell growth and reduces inflammation. Soldiers and healers in historical conflicts often relied on comfrey poultices to mend broken bones and bruises quickly, enabling injured combatants to return to battle sooner.

Calendula, or marigold, is another herb with a long history of medicinal use. Its antiseptic and anti-inflammatory qualities made it a staple in wartime first-aid kits. The bright yellow flowers of calendula were used as ointments and teas to clean wounds and soothe irritated skin, reducing the risk of infection.

Arnica Montana, often called mountain tobacco, is famous for its ability to reduce bruising and swelling. Healers would apply arnica compresses to soldiers' injuries, helping to alleviate pain and speed up recovery. Even today, arnica remains a popular choice among athletes and individuals seeking relief from sprains and muscle aches (*Our Ingredients*, 2022).

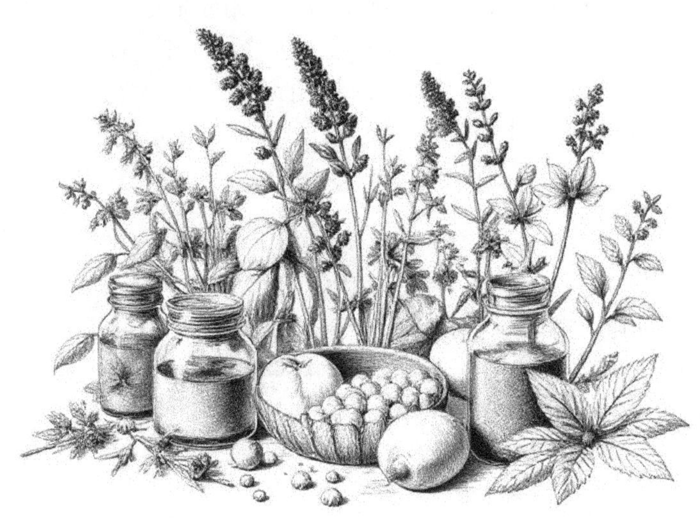

The resilience and ingenuity of humans in the face of adversity are highlighted through historical accounts of soldiers and healers employing these herbal remedies. During wars where conventional medical supplies were scarce or nonexistent, these natural treatments became indispensable. For instance, during the Napoleonic Wars, field surgeons frequently resorted to herbal poultices to care for the wounded when supplies dwindled. In such dire circumstances, the wisdom of traditional herbal practices shone through, proving their worth time and again.

Examining different cultures' approaches to healing war wounds using herbs reveals a universal reliance on available natural resources. Across continents and centuries, people have turned to the plants growing around them for healing. In Eastern Europe, for example, manuscripts dating back to the fourteenth century document the use of local herbs for medicinal purposes (Petran et al., 2020). Similarly, Native American tribes utilized plants like yarrow and echinacea to treat injuries sustained in battles, highlighting the shared human instinct to look to nature for solutions.

These traditional remedies, while born out of necessity, laid the groundwork for modern medical practices. The understanding gained from centuries of herbal use has inspired patient-centered recovery strategies today. Modern medicine continues to explore and incorporate compounds derived from these age-old remedies into treatments. Comfrey's allantoin is now found in numerous skincare products aimed at promoting healing and hydration. Arnica, too, is still widely used in topical applications for its analgesic properties.

Contemporary healthcare gently tips its hat to the past as more practitioners recognize the value of integrating herbal knowledge with modern science. While technological advancements have revolutionized medicine, the foundational principles learned from nature remain relevant. This merging of old and new exemplifies a holistic approach to health, emphasizing the importance of treating both the body and mind.

Moreover, understanding the cultural significance of herbal remedies can broaden perspectives and enhance empathy within healthcare systems. Knowing how different societies approach healing enriches our appreciation of the diversity of medical traditions and underscores the universality of seeking wellness in challenging times.

## Herbs Used for Anxiety During Ancient Natural Disasters

When natural disasters struck, ancient cultures leaned heavily on herbal remedies to manage the psychological trauma and anxiety that inevitably followed. Long before modern medicine came into the picture, herbs like lemon balm, valerian, and passionflower played a critical role in soothing frayed nerves and providing a much-needed respite from stress. These plants weren't just randomly plucked out of the earth; their calming attributes were well recognized, and ancient healers understood their significant impact on the nervous system.

Lemon balm, for instance, was celebrated for its gentle sedative properties. Healers used it to ease tension and promote relaxation, making it invaluable during crises when anxiety levels soared. Similarly, valerian root was esteemed for its ability to calm the mind and ensure restful sleep, which is vital for emotional stability. Passionflower also boasted anxiety-relieving qualities, often used in concoctions and teas to offer peace of mind and tranquility.

The availability of these herbal solutions meant that communities could address mental health effectively even amidst chaos. But these plants were not just ingested; they formed an integral part of cultural rituals. These rituals provided a structured way for individuals to cope with crises, allowing them to maintain a sense of community and continuity in turbulent times. When people gathered to prepare and consume these remedies, it fostered a collective healing environment. This communal approach not only targeted symptoms but also laid the foundation for comprehensive wellness, embracing both body and spirit.

There are numerous illustrative accounts of communities triumphantly utilizing herbal remedies, demonstrating resilience in the face of adversity. For example, historical records from regions prone to earthquakes show how entire villages relied on herbal concoctions to offer mental fortitude. By integrating these treatments into daily life, people could find balance and strength—a testament to human adaptability and resourcefulness.

Modern society, despite its reliance on synthetic medicines, still acknowledges the relevance of these ancient practices. In recent years, there's been a growing interest in reincorporating herbal remedies into mainstream treatments for anxiety and other mental health issues. Today's call for a more holistic approach mirrors the wisdom of our ancestors who recognized the power of plants. As modern science strives to understand the effects of these herbs, evidence mounts, supporting their efficacy and safety (Kenda et al., 2022).

Guidelines can assist individuals who seek to embrace herbal remedies as part of their coping strategies. These guidelines often emphasize consulting healthcare professionals before starting any herbal treatment, particularly for those already on medication. Understanding potential interactions is key, as herbs like St. John's Wort can interact with prescription drugs, altering their effectiveness (Baek et al., 2014). By being informed and cautious, individuals can safely integrate these traditional remedies into their lives.

The resurgence of interest in such therapies suggests not only their potent potential but also a desire to return to more natural, less invasive forms of healing. The enduring appeal of herbs like lemon balm, valerian, and passionflower lies in their capacity to provide comfort without the adverse side effects often associated with pharmaceuticals.

It's fascinating to note how ancient cultures, constrained by the technology of their time, developed sophisticated systems to combat psychological distress. Their reliance on nature's pharmacy highlights an intrinsic trust in the earth's resources—an ethos we seem to be returning to today. As ancient wisdom meets modern research, we find ourselves at a unique crossroads, one where the integration of these two worlds could pave the way for improved mental health strategies in our contemporary lives.

Taking cues from history doesn't mean forsaking advancements in medicine but enriching them. Blending the old with the new permits a wider range of therapeutic options, granting individuals the freedom to choose what works best for their mental health needs. Acknowledging the lessons of our predecessors allows us to adopt practices that align more closely with our natural rhythms and promote overall wellness.

## Emergency Herbal Remedies: Natural Solutions in Times of Crisis

In moments when modern medical supplies fall short, these herbal remedies provide vital support. The following instructions outline time-tested solutions—from healing wounds and reducing fevers to aiding digestion, easing anxiety, and preventing illness—that have sustained communities through challenging times.

### Wound Care

When injuries occur, natural remedies can accelerate healing and reduce inflammation.

#### Comfrey Poultice

For rapid wound healing and inflammation reduction.

**Ingredients:**

- Fresh comfrey leaves or dried comfrey herb

**Instructions:**

1. Crush fresh comfrey leaves into a paste, or steep dried leaves in hot water to create a poultice.
2. Apply directly to the wound and cover with a clean cloth.

**Contraindications:**

- For external use only. Do not apply on deep, open wounds or broken skin. Avoid ingesting comfrey, as it contains toxic compounds. Consult a healthcare professional if you are pregnant or breastfeeding.

## Calendula Ointment

For soothing minor cuts or scrapes and preventing infection.

**Ingredients:**

- Dried calendula flowers, olive oil, and beeswax

**Instructions:**

1. Infuse dried calendula flowers in olive oil for several weeks.
2. Strain the infusion and heat it with beeswax until melted.
3. Pour the mixture into a container and allow it to solidify.

**Contraindications:**

- Perform a patch test for skin sensitivity. Avoid use if you have an allergy to plants in the daisy family (ragweed).

## Arnica Compress

To reduce bruising or swelling and ease pain.

**Ingredients:**

- Arnica flowers or arnica tincture

**Instructions:**

1. Brew arnica flowers in hot water to create a compress or soak a cloth in diluted arnica tincture.
2. Apply the compress or cloth to bruises and swollen areas.

**Contraindications:**

- Do not use it on broken skin or open wounds. Arnica is for external use only and should be avoided by those allergic to it.

## Fever Reducers

Herbal remedies can help naturally lower body temperature and stimulate perspiration during fever.

### Yarrow Tea

To induce sweating and naturally reduce fever.

**Ingredients:**

- 1–2 tsp dried yarrow leaves and flowers
- Water

**Instructions:**

1. Steep tsp of dried yarrow in boiling water for 10–15 minutes.
2. Strain and drink the warm tea.

**Contraindications:**

- Avoid it if you are allergic to ragweed or similar plants. Pregnant women should use caution, as yarrow may stimulate uterine contractions.

### Sage Infusion

For its antiseptic and fever-reducing properties.

**Ingredients:**

- 1 tsp dried sage leaves
- Honey (optional)

**Instructions:**

1. Steep 1 tsp of dried sage in hot water for 10 minutes.
2. Optionally, add a touch of honey for flavor.

**Contraindications:**

- Large amounts of sage are not recommended for pregnant women. Use with caution if you have a history of seizures.

## Digestive Aids

When digestive discomfort arises, these remedies help soothe the stomach and promote healthy digestion.

### Chamomile Tea

For easing stomach discomfort and aiding digestion.

**Ingredients:**

- 1–2 tsp dried chamomile flowers
- Water
- Honey (optional)

**Instructions:**

1. Steep 1–2 tsp of dried chamomile flowers in boiling water for 5–10 minutes.
2. Strain and sweeten with honey if desired.

**Contraindications:**

- Those allergic to ragweed may experience reactions. Consult your healthcare provider if pregnant or breastfeeding.

### Ginger Tincture

For soothing nausea and promoting smooth digestion.

**Ingredients:**

- Fresh ginger root
- Alcohol (vodka or brandy)

**Instructions:**

1. Chop fresh ginger root and submerge in alcohol in a sealed jar.
2. Let it steep for at least two weeks, shaking the jar daily.
3. Strain and store in a bottle.

**Contraindications:**

- Use with caution if you are on blood thinners or have gallstones or ulcers. Pregnant women should consult a healthcare professional before use.

## Anxiety Relief

Herbal remedies can help calm the mind and ease anxiety during stressful times.

### Lemon Balm Tea

For calming the mind and reducing anxiety.

**Ingredients:**

- 1–2 tsp fresh lemon balm leaves or dried lemon balm

**Instructions:**

1. Steep 1–2 tsp of lemon balm in hot water for 10 minutes.
2. Strain and enjoy the soothing tea.

**Contraindications:**

- Generally safe; consult a healthcare provider if you have thyroid issues or are pregnant.

### Valerian Root Extract

For promoting relaxation and supporting restful sleep.

**Ingredients:**

- Dried valerian root

- Alcohol or glycerin

**Instructions:**

1. Soak dried valerian root in alcohol or glycerin for 4–6 weeks and then strain.
2. Use a small dose mixed with water.

**Contraindications:**

- May cause drowsiness; avoid operating heavy machinery after use. Not recommended for pregnant or breastfeeding women and may interact with sedatives or alcohol.

## Preventive Measures

Preventive herbal remedies help protect your environment and overall health by warding off pathogens.

### Herbal Air Purifiers—Thyme and Rosemary Tincture

For purifying the air and providing antimicrobial benefits.

**Ingredients:**

- Fresh thyme and rosemary
- Alcohol

**Instructions:**

1. Fill a jar with fresh thyme and rosemary.
2. Cover the herbs completely with alcohol and let the mixture steep for 4 weeks.
3. Use drops in water or as a room spray.

**Contraindications:**

- Do not ingest in large amounts. Use caution if you are pregnant or if the remedy is to be used around children.

Each of these remedies reflects centuries of herbal wisdom, offering practical solutions when conventional resources are limited. Always consult a healthcare professional before use, especially if you have pre-existing conditions or are pregnant, breastfeeding, or taking other medications. Embrace these natural methods to support healing and maintain well-being even in challenging times.

## Bringing It All Together

Throughout history, herbal remedies have played vital roles during times of crisis, like the Black Plague. These natural solutions were not just random choices; they represented a deep knowledge of plant properties that could soothe symptoms and bring some relief amidst the chaos. By using herbs such as yarrow, sage, and chamomile, communities managed to tackle fevers and inflammations, showing an impressive understanding of how these plants work.

This chapter shed light on how the creative use of herbal tinctures helped purify the air, offering an early example of preventive healthcare. Such reliance on nature's offerings highlights the adaptability and resilience of people who turned to what was accessible when traditional medicine couldn't keep up.

The lessons from such historical practices are valuable today. Preserving the knowledge of medicinal plants remains crucial, especially in times when modern resources might be stretched thin. By learning from these past experiences, we understand the significance of integrating preventive strategies into our healthcare approach. Moreover, trusting local healers and herbalists can strengthen community health responses.

Embracing holistic methods does not mean leaving science behind but rather enriching it with age-old wisdom. The chapter encourages one to reflect on how blending traditional and modern practices leads to a more comprehensive health strategy, benefiting both individuals and entire communities.

# Chapter 4: Everyday Ailments and Ancient Solutions

Dealing with everyday ailments often sends us rushing to the medicine cabinet, but several ancient remedies promise relief, using nature's own pharmacy. These time-honored solutions have been part of human history long before the advent of modern medicine.

From soothing sore throats with honey to treating digestive issues with peppermint and improving skin conditions with aloe vera, ancient civilizations tapped into the natural world to heal common discomforts. The allure of these remedies lies not only in their historical roots but also in the fact that they harness simple, accessible ingredients. By turning our gaze back to these past practices, we might uncover some hidden treasures that can complement our contemporary health routines.

In this chapter, you'll journey through time as we explore the fascinating ways traditional herbal treatments have addressed everyday health issues. We'll examine how ancient Greeks, Egyptians, and Romans utilized honey for its antimicrobial properties, providing natural relief for throat soreness. Then, we'll take a look at peppermint, a fragrant herb prized by ancient cultures for its calming effects on the digestive system, which now finds validation in scientific studies. Lastly, you'll discover the secrets of aloe vera, celebrated for centuries for its ability to soothe skin irritations and encourage healing.

Each section reveals the historical significance, practical applications, and modern-day validations of these herbal treasures. Through this exploration, you will gain insight into how these age-old remedies continue to offer simple yet effective pathways toward better health.

## Honey's Role in Soothing Sore Throats

Honey, often referred to as "liquid gold," has been cherished throughout history for its medicinal properties, particularly in soothing sore throats. Ancient cultures from Egypt and Greece to India recognized honey not only as a sweetener but also as a therapeutic agent. Its rich antimicrobial properties were well-documented in various traditional medical systems, including Ayurveda and Islamic medicine.

The use of honey as a remedy dates back thousands of years. The ancient Egyptians frequently included honey in their medicinal recipes, using it for ailments ranging from throat irritations to infections (Eteraf-Oskouei & Najafi, 2012). Similarly, the Greeks valued honey's healing abilities. Hippocrates, one of the most influential figures in the history of medicine, advocated using honey mixed with water to ease a sore throat (Eteraf-Oskouei & Najafi, 2012). The idea that honey held powerful healing properties pervaded many ancient texts and practices, emphasizing its role in treating both internal and external maladies.

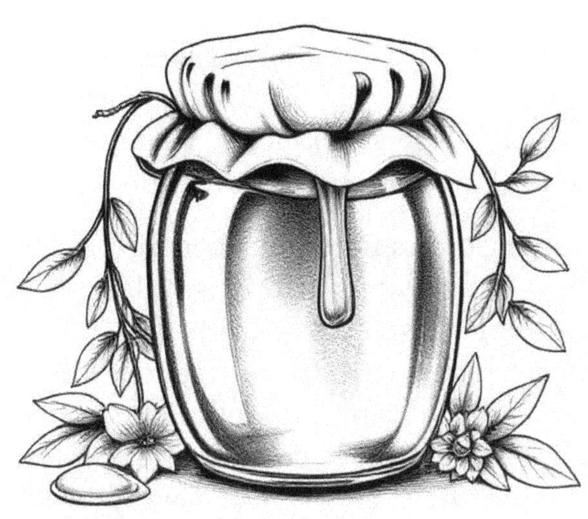

In contemporary times, modern science has validated many of these traditional uses of honey. Research supports honey's efficacy as a natural cough suppressant, often surpassing synthetic remedies. Studies highlight how honey can effectively reduce cough frequency and severity, providing greater relief than some over-the-counter options (Mandal & Mandal, 2011). This effectiveness is largely due to honey's ability to coat the throat, offering immediate soothing through its viscous texture while its natural antioxidants and bioactive compounds promote healing.

For those looking to incorporate honey into their wellness routine today, there are several practical methods. The simplest approach is to mix honey with warm water. This age-old combination is known to soothe an irritated throat upon contact. Beyond water, adding honey to herbal teas enhances the beverage's therapeutic potential, especially when combined with herbs like chamomile or ginger known for their additional health benefits. Adding a splash of lemon juice not only complements honey's flavor but also introduces vitamin C and other antibacterial properties to the mixture.

While honey offers numerous benefits, it's essential to be aware of safety considerations. Most notably, honey should never be given to infants under one year of age due to the risk of botulism, a serious illness caused by bacteria that may be present in honey (Mandal & Mandal, 2011). Adults and older children, however, can generally enjoy honey safely, although it's always wise to ensure it is genuine and raw, as processed honey might lose some beneficial properties.

## Peppermint for Treating Digestive Issues

Since ancient times, peppermint has enjoyed a reputation for calming troubled stomachs. In the bustling markets of ancient Greece and Rome, where food was abundant and rich, peppermint stood out not only for its refreshing flavor but also for its ability to alleviate digestive discomforts like bloating and gas. It was so esteemed that texts from these eras point to its inclusion in diets as both a culinary spice and therapeutic ally.

The Greeks would often use peppermint after meals to help with digestion, while Romans incorporated it into their feasts to counteract any potential aftermath of indulgence. This historical backdrop highlights how deeply intertwined peppermint has been with dietary practices specifically aimed at promoting digestive health.

Fast forward to modern times, and science has stepped in to validate what the ancients seemed to have known intuitively. Multiple scientific studies have turned their focus toward peppermint, particularly its active compound menthol, which is noted for relaxing the muscles of the gastrointestinal tract.

These findings are crucial because they provide a scientific basis for using peppermint in relieving conditions such as irritable bowel syndrome (IBS). IBS, characterized by symptoms like cramping, abdominal pain, bloating, gas, and diarrhea or constipation, affects millions worldwide. Here, peppermint oil capsules have emerged as a popular remedy due to menthol's capability to soothe intestinal spasms, thus offering a natural alternative to conventional medications (Chumpitazi et al., 2018).

For those seeking practical ways to incorporate peppermint into their wellness regimen, this versatile herb doesn't disappoint. Peppermint teas are a delightful starting point. A simple brew made from dried peppermint leaves can be soothing after a heavy meal, easing indigestion and providing gentle relief from stomach discomforts.

Additionally, peppermint-infused oils, either in capsule form or as a topical application on the abdomen, offer another avenue for relief. These methods are not only accessible but can be seamlessly integrated into daily routines for those looking to embrace herbal remedies. It's important to remember, though, that consistency and moderation are key when incorporating peppermint into your routine.

Like all remedies, peppermint comes with a set of considerations. People with gastroesophageal reflux disease (GERD) should exercise caution when using peppermint. Its muscle-relaxing effects, which are beneficial in many contexts, can paradoxically exacerbate GERD symptoms by causing the lower esophageal sphincter to relax, potentially leading to increased acid reflux. Therefore, individuals with GERD need to consult with healthcare professionals before integrating peppermint into their treatment plans (*Peppermint Oil*, 2020). Additionally, adhering to recommended dosages is imperative since excessive consumption might lead to unwanted side effects such as heartburn or allergic reactions.

On the label of many peppermint products, you'll find suggestions on dosage and usage tailored to different health needs. Reading and following these instructions is an essential practice. If you're preparing homemade remedies, striking the right balance in concentration ensures effectiveness without overwhelming the body. Whether it's a steaming cup of peppermint tea or a few drops of infused oil, each application provides a unique method to harness the power of peppermint while respecting its potency.

## Aloe Vera for Skin Conditions

Aloe vera, often referred to as the "plant of immortality," has a long-standing reputation for its remarkable skin benefits. This succulent plant has been cherished since ancient Egyptian times for its ability to promote skin health and facilitate healing processes. The Egyptians included it in their beauty regimes, attributing their radiant skin to its soothing properties (Hekmatpou et al., 2017). This admiration for aloe vera has endured through the centuries, as it's no longer folklore but supported by empirical research that highlights its efficacy for various skin conditions.

Modern science confirms what the ancients suspected: aloe vera is excellent for enhancing wound healing and reducing inflammation (Surjushe et al., 2008). It's particularly beneficial for individuals dealing with conditions like psoriasis and eczema. The transparent gel within aloe leaves includes compounds such as glucomannan, which stimulates fibroblast growth and collagen production, essential for skin repair and regeneration (Surjushe et al., 2008). These properties make it invaluable for those looking to manage chronic skin disorders or everyday irritations.

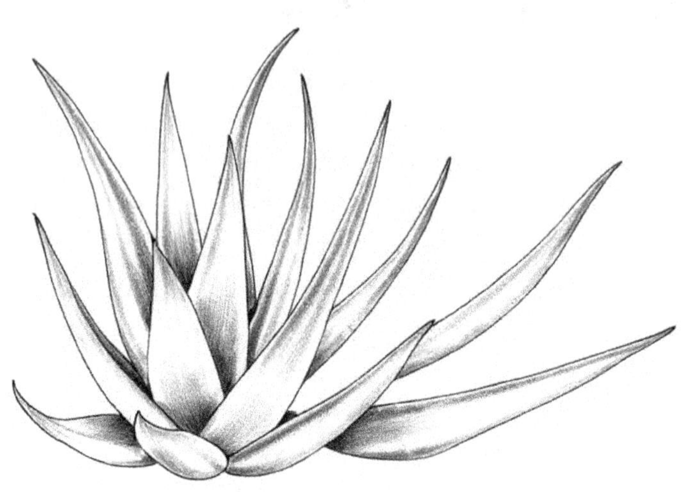

Aloe vera can become a staple in your home remedies for natural skincare. Preparing fresh aloe gel is straightforward; simply slice open a leaf and scoop out the clear substance inside. This gel can be applied directly to the skin to soothe conditions, burns, or cuts. Additionally, you can create aloe-infused lotions or creams by mixing the gel with other natural ingredients such as coconut oil or lavender essential oil for added benefits.

Growing your own aloe plant at home is both practical and rewarding. Aloe vera thrives in warm, dry environments and requires minimal care, making it an ideal choice for even the most novice gardeners. Place it in a sunny spot, water sparingly, and watch it flourish. Having access to fresh aloe ensures that you're using the purest form of the plant, free from any additives or preservatives that might be found in commercial products.

However, while aloe vera is generally safe for topical use, you must be aware of the potential allergic reactions it may cause. Some individuals may experience redness or irritation upon application. To mitigate this risk, it's best to perform a patch test before full application. Apply a small amount of gel to a discreet area and observe if any adverse reactions occur over 24 hours. If your skin responds well, you can proceed confidently with broader use.

Ensuring the purity of your aloe vera source is crucial. Opt for organic aloe products when purchasing commercially prepared gels or creams to avoid chemicals or synthetic additives. Additionally, seeking professional advice may be worthwhile for those with severe skin conditions. Dermatologists can provide expert guidance on incorporating aloe vera into a broader treatment plan, ensuring its benefits are maximized safely and effectively.

## Time-Tested Herbal Remedies: Garlic, Turmeric, Chamomile, and More

Homeopathy extends beyond the known remedies of honey, peppermint, and aloe vera. Looking to other ancient wisdom can lead to simple recipes that tackle a spectrum of ailments. For example, ginger has been used for centuries to address nausea and digestive issues. An everyday remedy involves preparing ginger tea by boiling fresh ginger slices in water for ten minutes and then straining and adding honey for flavor. This soothing tea can be consumed whenever you feel nauseous or uneasy, providing relief from stomach discomfort.

Garlic is another powerful ancient remedy, renowned for its immune-boosting properties. A popular method to incorporate garlic for wellness is to prepare garlic-infused oil. Slice several cloves of garlic and gently simmer them in olive oil over low heat for about 30 minutes. Once cool, strain out the garlic and store the oil in a glass jar. This infused oil can be used in cooking to add flavor while harnessing health benefits or applied topically to minor cuts to help prevent infection.

Turmeric, known for its anti-inflammatory and antioxidant properties, is another staple in ancient medicine systems. One effective way to utilize turmeric is by creating a golden milk drink. Simply warm a cup of milk or dairy alternative and whisk in one tsp of turmeric powder, a pinch of black pepper, and honey to taste. This warming tonic can help reduce inflammation in the body and is especially comforting before bed.

Chamomile, cherished for its calming effects, can be transformed into a comforting chamomile tea. Steep dried chamomile flowers in hot water for five minutes and then strain. This tea serves as an excellent nighttime beverage, promoting relaxation and preparation for restful sleep. It's a natural remedy for anxiety and insomnia, blending well with honey for added sweetness and soothing properties.

For skin ailments beyond what aloe vera addresses, consider using tea tree oil, which is known for its antiseptic qualities. To create a simple tea tree oil treatment, mix a few drops of tea tree oil with a carrier oil such as coconut or jojoba. Apply this blend to areas affected by acne or minor cuts. The mixture can help reduce the appearance of blemishes while preventing infection, reflecting ancient practices of using herbal oils for beauty and health.

Cinnamon, revered for its antioxidant and anti-inflammatory qualities, is another ingredient that can be incorporated into a wellness routine. One easily prepared remedy is cinnamon water. Boil a few cinnamon sticks in water and then let it cool before straining it. This tasty drink can help regulate blood sugar levels and may support digestion. A touch of honey can both enhance the flavor and add a soothing effect for those suffering from throat irritation.

Lemon and garlic together offer a delightful and healthful infusion. Combining freshly squeezed lemon juice with crushed garlic and honey creates a powerful immune-boosting tonic. Mix these in a glass of warm water and drink it in the morning for an energizing start to the day. This simple recipe leverages garlic's antimicrobial properties while using the vitamin C in lemon to support overall health.

Hibiscus flowers, often used in ancient cultures, provide more than just beauty. Create hibiscus tea by steeping dried hibiscus flowers in boiling water for ten minutes. This vibrant drink can help lower blood pressure and improve heart health. Sweetening it with honey offers additional health benefits and makes for a refreshing beverage on warm days.

Consider using chamomile in another form like preparing a calming herbal bath. Add a few handfuls of dried chamomile flowers to a muslin bag and steep in warm bathwater. This relaxing soak can soothe irritated skin and calm the mind, making it a wonderful addition to the self-care routine.

Basil, celebrated in various ancient cultures, offers a robust flavor and numerous health advantages. Create basil water by steeping fresh basil leaves in hot water for several hours. This infusion provides hydration while aiding digestion and can also be sweetened with a touch of honey or mixed into smoothies for a fresh flavor.

For summer headaches or migration relief, a refreshing mint and cucumber cooler can be effective. Blend fresh mint leaves with peeled cucumber and a sprinkle of sea salt. Mix with chilled water and strain for a revitalizing drink that hydrates while soothing headaches and tension, embodying the spirit of herbal remedies used throughout history.

Through these simple recipes, the ancient knowledge of herbal remedies becomes accessible for anyone looking to enhance their wellness routine. These ingredients not only provide effective natural relief but also celebrate the wisdom of generations before us. Embracing these ancient solutions promotes a holistic approach to health, blending the best of historical practices with modern needs. Each homemade remedy forms a bridge connecting the past and present, reaffirming the profound effectiveness of nature's bounty in our everyday lives. As we incorporate these wellness recipes, we can take charge of our health journeys—one soothing concoction at a time.

## Timeless Tonic Recipes: Harnessing Ancient Wisdom for Modern Wellness

Dealing with everyday ailments often sends us rushing to the medicine cabinet—but nature's own pharmacy offers time-honored solutions that have soothed discomforts for centuries. The following section presents a collection of practical recipes inspired by ancient wisdom.

### Everyday Practical Remedies With Minimal Ingredients

The following recipes present a collection of practical remedies inspired by ancient wisdom.

#### Honey Throat Soother

Let the ancient power of honey work its magic, coating and calming your irritated throat with every soothing sip.

**Ingredients:**

- 1 tbsp raw honey
- 1 cup warm water
- Optional: A squeeze of fresh lemon juice

**Instructions:**

1. In a cup, combine the raw honey with warm water.
2. Stir until the honey is fully dissolved.
3. Add lemon juice if desired and stir again.
4. Sip slowly, allowing the viscous mixture to coat your throat.

**Contraindications:**

- Do not give honey to infants under one year of age.
- Individuals allergic to honey should avoid this remedy.
- Consult a healthcare professional if you have any concerns.

## Peppermint Digestive Tea

Let the refreshing power of peppermint ease your stomach, calming cramps and promoting smooth digestion with every revitalizing sip.

**Ingredients:**

- 1–2 tsp dried peppermint leaves
- 1 cup boiling water

**Instructions:**

1. Place the dried peppermint leaves in a teapot or heatproof cup.
2. Pour one cup of boiling water over the leaves.

3. Steep for 10 minutes.
4. Strain the tea into a cup and enjoy warm.

**Contraindications:**

- Those with gastroesophageal reflux disease (GERD) should use caution.
- Consult a healthcare professional if you are unsure about its use.

### Aloe Vera Skin Soother

Let the cooling power of aloe vera soothe skin irritation and promote healing with every gentle application.

**Ingredients:**

- Fresh aloe vera gel (extracted from one aloe leaf)

**Instructions:**

1. Slice open an aloe leaf and scoop out the clear gel.
2. Apply the gel directly to the affected skin area.
3. Leave it on for 15–20 minutes before rinsing it off gently.

**Contraindications:**

- Perform a patch test first to check for allergic reactions.
- Avoid use if you have a known allergy to aloe vera.

## Ginger Tea

Let the warming essence of ginger tea invigorate your body with its time-tested, soothing properties that help with digestion and nausea.

**Ingredients:**

- 1-inch piece of fresh ginger, sliced thinly
- 1 cup water
- Honey to taste (optional)

**Instructions:**

1. Bring the water to a boil.
2. Add the ginger slices and simmer for 10 minutes.
3. Strain the tea into a cup.
4. Stir in honey, if desired, and drink warm.

**Contraindications:**

- Use with caution if you have gallstones or ulcers.
- Consult a healthcare professional if you're pregnant or on certain medications.

## Garlic-Infused Oil

Let the robust flavor of garlic-infused oil work its magic on your immune system, unleashing potent antimicrobial benefits with every golden drop.

**Ingredients:**

- 4 garlic cloves, crushed
- ½ cup olive oil

**Instructions:**

1. Crush the garlic cloves and let them rest for 5 minutes to activate the allicin.
2. In a small saucepan, combine the garlic with olive oil over low heat for 15 minutes—do not let it boil.
3. Remove from heat and allow the oil to cool.
4. Strain the oil into a clean glass jar.

**Contraindications:**

- May cause gastrointestinal discomfort in sensitive individuals.
- Not recommended for those with garlic allergies.

## Turmeric Golden Milk

Let the warm embrace of turmeric golden milk soothe your body, blending ancient spice with modern wellness for anti-inflammatory benefits in every comforting cup.

**Ingredients:**

- 1 cup milk or a dairy alternative
- 1 tsp turmeric powder
- A pinch of black pepper
- Honey to taste

**Instructions:**

1. Warm the milk in a saucepan over medium heat.
2. Whisk in the turmeric powder and black pepper until well combined.

3. Remove from heat, add honey for sweetness, and stir thoroughly.
4. Enjoy warm.

**Contraindications:**

- Avoid if you have a turmeric allergy.
- Consult a healthcare professional if on blood-thinning medication.

## Chamomile Tea

Let the gentle power of chamomile tea calm your mind and ease your stomach with every soothing sip.

**Ingredients:**

- 1–2 tsp dried chamomile flowers
- 1 cup boiling water
- Honey (optional)

**Instructions:**

1. Place the chamomile flowers in a teapot or heatproof cup.
2. Pour boiling water over the flowers and steep for 5–10 minutes.
3. Strain the tea into a cup and add honey if desired.

**Contraindications:**

- Check for allergies, particularly if sensitive to ragweed.
- Use cautiously if pregnant or breastfeeding; consult your healthcare provider.

## Tea Tree Oil Treatment

Let the antiseptic strength of tea tree oil help cleanse and protect your skin from blemishes and minor cuts with every careful application.

### Ingredients:

- 3–4 drops tea tree oil
- 1 tsp carrier oil (such as coconut or jojoba)

### Instructions:

1. Mix the tea tree oil with the carrier oil thoroughly.
2. Apply a small amount of the mixture to the affected area.
3. Repeat 1–2 times daily as needed.

### Contraindications:

- Do not use undiluted tea tree oil on the skin.
- Perform a patch test prior to full application.
- Avoid using on broken skin.

## Cinnamon Water

Let the warm spice of cinnamon water invigorate your system with its subtle, comforting flavor.

### Ingredients:

- 2 cinnamon sticks
- 1 cup water
- Honey to taste (optional)

**Instructions:**

1. Boil the water with the cinnamon sticks for 10 minutes.
2. Allow the mixture to cool slightly and then strain it into a cup.
3. Stir in honey if desired and drink it warm or at room temperature.

**Contraindications:**

- Avoid excessive consumption.
- Consult a healthcare professional if pregnant or managing blood sugar issues.

### Lemon Garlic Tonic

Let the zesty blend of lemon, garlic, and honey create a revitalizing tonic that boosts immunity and energizes your day from the very first sip.

**Ingredients:**

- 1 lemon (juiced)
- 2 garlic cloves, crushed
- 1 tbsp raw honey
- 1 cup warm water

**Instructions:**

1. In a cup, combine the lemon juice, crushed garlic, and raw honey
2. Add warm water and stir well until the honey dissolves.

3. Drink immediately for a potent immune boost.

**Contraindications:**

- Not recommended for individuals with garlic allergies.
- Use caution if you suffer from acid reflux or a sensitive stomach.

## Hibiscus Tea

Let the vibrant power of hibiscus tea refresh and rejuvenate you with its tangy, colorful infusion that supports heart health and blood pressure.

**Ingredients:**

- 1–2 tsp dried hibiscus flowers
- 1 cup boiling water
- Honey to taste (optional)

**Instructions:**

1. Place the dried hibiscus flowers in a teapot.
2. Pour boiling water over them and steep for 10 minutes.
3. Strain the tea into a cup, add honey if desired, and serve warm or chilled.

**Contraindications:**

- May lower blood pressure; consult a healthcare professional if you have hypotension or are on antihypertensive medication.

## Chamomile Herbal Bath

Let a chamomile herbal bath wash away stress and calm irritated skin with its gentle, fragrant touch.

### Ingredients:

- 1 cup dried chamomile flowers
- A muslin bag
- Warm bathwater

### Instructions:

1. Place the dried chamomile flowers into a muslin bag and tie it securely.
2. Add the bag to a warm bath and allow it to steep for 20 minutes.
3. Soak in the bath and enjoy the calming effects.

### Contraindications:

- Generally safe; perform a patch test if you have sensitive skin or known allergies.

## Basil Water

Let the aromatic essence of basil water refresh and hydrate your body and aid in digestion with each revitalizing sip.

### Ingredients:

- A handful of fresh basil leaves
- 1 liter water

**Instructions:**

1. Add the fresh basil leaves to the water.
2. Allow the mixture to steep in the refrigerator for several hours.
3. Strain and serve chilled.

**Contraindications:**

- Generally safe; consult if you have any known allergies to basil.

### Mint and Cucumber Cooler

For a refreshing pick-me-up and headache relief, let the crisp combination of mint and cucumber create a revitalizing cooler that hydrates and soothes tension.

**Ingredients:**

- A handful of fresh mint leaves
- ½ cucumber, peeled and chopped
- A pinch of sea salt
- 2 cups chilled water

**Instructions:**

1. Blend the mint leaves and chopped cucumber with a pinch of sea salt until smooth.
2. Add the chilled water and blend briefly to combine.
3. Strain the mixture if desired and serve over ice.

**Contraindications:**

- Generally safe; consult a healthcare professional if you have known allergies to mint or cucumber.

## Bringing It All Together

In this chapter, we've delved into the world of traditional herbal treatments for everyday ailments, highlighting some natural remedies that have stood the test of time. From honey's soothing abilities for a sore throat to peppermint's knack for easing digestive woes and aloe vera's healing touch for skin conditions, plants offer simple yet effective ways to enhance our wellness routine. It's fascinating how modern science backs up what ancient cultures have known all along, giving us even more reason to explore these time-honored remedies.

As we incorporate these herbal treasures into our lives, it's important to do so thoughtfully. Whether you're stirring honey into your tea, sipping on peppermint brews, or applying fresh aloe gel, keep in mind the importance of understanding both benefits and precautions. Consulting with healthcare professionals can be helpful, especially if you have pre-existing conditions or specific health concerns. Embracing these natural remedies is about blending tradition with personal care, ensuring we enjoy several ancient remedies that promise the best of both worlds safely and effectively.

# Chapter 5: Emotional and Spiritual Healing

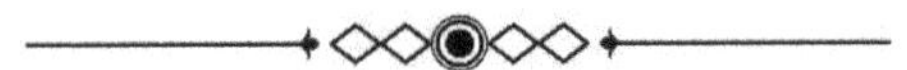

Healing the mind and spirit by tapping into nature's bounty is a practice that has long fascinated humanity. From ancient civilizations to modern wellness routines, herbs have played a special role in promoting mental and spiritual well-being. In times when medical knowledge was limited and pharmaceuticals were mere figments of imagination, people turned to the world around them for solace and healing.

Herbs like chamomile, lavender, and sage emerged as powerful allies in this quest. These humble plants were more than just remedies; they became woven into the very fabric of cultural and spiritual practices. Using what was readily available, our ancestors honed ways to soothe stress and cultivate inner peace, leaving behind traditions that echo in today's holistic approaches.

As we journey through this chapter, we'll explore how these three herbs worked their magic in the realms of emotional and spiritual healing. We begin with chamomile, an herb known for its calming effects since ancient times, helping troubled minds find tranquility and facilitating restful sleep. Then, we'll move to lavender's sweet aroma and its knack for easing tension and encouraging relaxation. Beyond its soothing properties, lavender's historical use in fostering peace and enhancing spiritual clarity will also come to light. Lastly, we'll look at sage, whose smudging rituals carry spiritual significance, purifying environments and inviting positive energy.

This chapter shines a light on the ancient wisdom surrounding these remarkable herbs and illustrates their enduring impact on well-being.

## The Calming Effects of Chamomile

Chamomile has been cherished for centuries across various cultures as a comforting and calming herb. Its historical roots trace back to ancient civilizations, where it was commonly employed in bedtime rituals. Imagine living in a time when modern pharmaceuticals were not an option—people turned to nature's remedies to soothe their minds.

In societies such as Ancient Egypt and Rome, chamomile was frequently used to alleviate anxiety and induce relaxation, particularly before sleep. This practice was based on both tradition and the observable effects of the plant. Chamomile tea or infusions became a staple in households, serving as a gentle lullaby that eased individuals into restful slumbers.

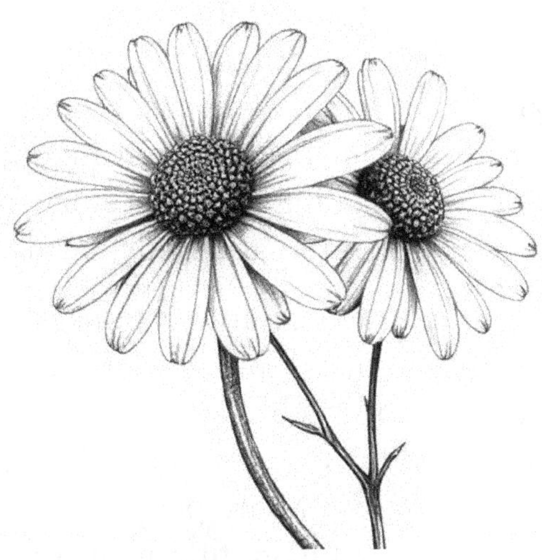

In today's world, scientific research has peeled back the layers of the folklore surrounding chamomile to reveal its biological secrets. Modern studies have validated what our ancestors seemed to understand intuitively: chamomile truly does help reduce anxiety and improve sleep quality.

Its magic lies in compounds like apigenin, a bioactive component known to bind to certain receptors in the brain, which may decrease anxiety and foster better sleep (Gupta, 2010). These findings underscore chamomile's relevance in contemporary mental health practices, offering a natural alternative for those who prefer botanical solutions over synthetic medications.

Another noteworthy aspect of chamomile is its anti-inflammatory properties, which play a crucial role in promoting overall psychological stability. We often forget that mental well-being is intricately linked to physical health. When the body is free from inflammation, there is a noticeable improvement in mood and emotional balance. Chamomile contains essential oils that possess anti-inflammatory characteristics, contributing to general wellness and indirectly supporting mental health (Sah et al., 2022). It's fascinating how this small, daisy-like flower can influence both mind and body harmony.

In terms of its practical applications, chamomile offers numerous possibilities that go beyond traditional tea. Sure, a warm cup of chamomile tea remains a popular choice for winding down after a hectic day, but let's explore its versatility. Many people enjoy experimenting with chamomile by integrating it into recipes combined with other herbs. A simple yet delightful recipe could involve infusing chamomile with mint and a touch of lavender, creating a soothing herbal blend perfect for stress relief. Herbalists suggest that such combinations can magnify chamomile's relaxing effects, capitalizing on each plant's unique properties.

Additionally, chamomile's role extends to more creative uses, like homemade bath soaks or herbal pillows, providing comfort through aroma therapy. Designing personalized blends can become a form of mindful practice, allowing individuals to connect with nature and their senses. This adds a personal touch to self-care routines, turning everyday activities into moments of tranquility.

## Lavender's Role in Sleep and Relaxation

Lavender, a beloved herb throughout the ages, has long been associated with enhancing sleep and relaxation. The ancient Romans were among the first to recognize its calming properties. They commonly used lavender in their baths to create tranquil atmospheres, which they believed helped soothe both body and mind, preparing them for restful sleep. Lavender's place in matrimonial customs also highlights its associative role in fostering peace and calmness, both crucial elements in building harmonious familial bonds.

Today, the science behind lavender's historical reputation is becoming clearer. Modern research confirms what ancient civilizations believed: lavender's aroma can be a powerful ally against insomnia. Studies demonstrate that inhaling lavender oil before bed significantly improves sleep quality by reducing restlessness and aiding in more consistent sleep patterns. This is linked to lavender's ability to decrease levels of cortisol, the stress hormone that can interfere with sleep, thus establishing a biological foundation for its use as a natural sleep enhancer (Yogi et al., 2021).

Lavender-infused products have gained popularity in recent years as effective tools for incorporating this knowledge into daily life. Essential oil blends, often combined with other calming scents like chamomile or bergamot, are widely used in diffusers as part of bedtime rituals.

Sachets filled with dried lavender flowers are another common method; when slipped under pillows or placed around bedrooms, their subtle scent can naturally enhance the sleeping environment without relying on pharmaceutical aids. These practical applications highlight how seamlessly lavender can integrate into modern lifestyles while maintaining its traditional roles.

Beyond aiding sleep, lavender holds a revered place in spiritual practices. Its use in purification rituals dates back centuries when it used to be employed to cleanse spaces and elevate spiritual clarity. Many contemporary holistic wellness practitioners continue to use lavender for these purposes, valuing its ability to support environmental and mental purity. It serves as a bridge connecting modern spiritual seekers with ancient practices, reinforcing its significance in both personal and communal well-being.

Several accessible methods can help individuals incorporate lavender into their relaxation routines. One practical application involves creating a soothing bedtime ritual. Individuals might consider applying a blend of lavender essential oil diluted in a carrier oil to pulse points such as the temples and wrists before bed. Alternatively, adding a few drops of lavender oil to bath water can provide calming effects similar to a Roman bath experience, relaxing muscles and quieting the mind after a long day.

Another simple yet effective technique is to use a lavender pillow spray. Spritzing it lightly over bedding shortly before retiring can subtly infuse the sleep environment with a calming aroma. Over time, such rituals can become comforting habits that signal the body to wind down, aligning bedtime preparation with the body's natural circadian rhythms.

## Spiritual Use of Sage in Purification

Sage as a sacred plant within numerous cultural rituals has an intriguing history that stretches far back into antiquity. Its primary use in smudging ceremonies has made it a cornerstone of spiritual purification and healing practices.

Smudging refers to the burning of sage bundles to cleanse spaces, bodies, or objects, driving away negative energy and fostering spiritual hygiene. This age-old practice is especially prominent among Native American cultures, where it serves not only as a method of purification but also as a pathway for connecting with ancestral wisdom.

The importance of sage in these rituals transcends its role as a mere aromatic herb. The smoke from burning sage is believed to convey prayers to heaven and prevent negative energies from taking hold, creating a spiritually hygienic environment. Such practices can be seen in ceremonies where the smoke is directed around individuals, homes, or sacred items, believed to purify them before engaging in spiritual activities. The deeply rooted tradition of using sage to maintain emotional balance highlights its historical significance across many societies (Nguyen, 2024).

Modern scientific studies have begun to support some of these traditional uses by highlighting sage's antibacterial properties. When burned, sage releases ions, which reduce stress and improve mood levels. These ions are thought to aid in dispelling negative emotions, thus contributing to a person's mental clarity and peace of mind.

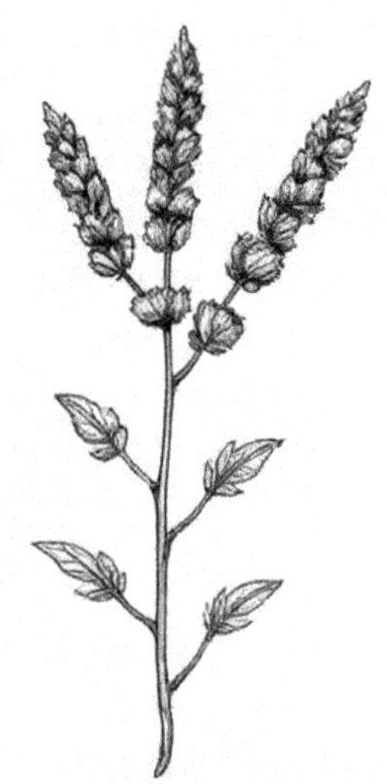

Practicing aromatherapy with sage has been shown to alleviate anxiety, making it a valuable tool for emotional healing. As people burn sage, the ritualistic act in itself becomes a form of meditation, helping individuals ground themselves and focus their intentions on positivity and replenishment (Larkin, 2023).

For those interested in incorporating sage into their own routines, knowing how to perform a smudging ceremony can be beneficial. It involves a few simple steps. First, one must gather a bundle of sage, ensuring it is sourced ethically and sustainably. Next, light the tip of the bundle until it begins to smolder, producing thick smoke. Then, gently fan this smoke over the intended areas, whether it's your room or around a person's body, utilizing a feather or even your hand. During this process, focus on your purpose, whether it's clearing negativity, protecting against future harm, or inviting peace and tranquility. Once complete, extinguish the bundle and store it safely for future use. This practice encourages mindfulness and offers a ritualistic approach to well-being.

In addition to its spiritual applications, sage has played a significant cultural role in various traditions beyond the Native American context. In European folklore, sage was believed to grant wisdom and longevity and often appeared in medicinal recipes aimed at improving mental clarity and memory.

Sage's reputation as a powerful plant extends into other indigenous communities, such as those of the Ancient Romans, who valued it for its purported health benefits, including digestive and cognitive support. These ancient civilizations recognized something profound in sage, attributing mystical properties to it that underscored its versatile nature.

Sage not only offers cleansing and mental clarity but also connects the past and present, linking us with our roots through its continuous use in spiritual practices. Whether used for smudging, sharing wisdom, or simply bolstering one's spirit, sage remains a timeless tool embraced by many around the world.

Emphasizing the versatility of sage in spiritual and emotional practices helps illustrate why it endures as a staple of holistic wellness. It's a conduit that bridges the gap between the tangible and the ethereal, offering a means of communicating with elements of the unseen world.

Moreover, understanding sage's antibacterial and calming properties expands its relevance, providing modern practitioners with diverse ways to engage with this venerated herb. Embracing sage in this manner ensures that it continues to empower those seeking harmony both within themselves and their surroundings, resonating through time as a beacon of purification and peace (Nguyen, 2024).

## Sacred Serenity Recipes: Timeless Herbal Formulations for Mind and Spirit

Healing the mind and spirit by tapping into nature's bounty is a practice that has long fascinated humanity. Drawing on traditions from ancient civilizations, these recipes offer simple, practical ways to incorporate herbal remedies into your daily routine for relaxation, better sleep, and enhanced mood.

### Simple Remedies for Nurturing the Body, Mind, and Spirit

These simple remedies, rooted in ancient wisdom, offer natural solutions to nurture your body, calm your mind, and elevate your spirit, helping you achieve balance and wellness in your daily life.

### Chamomile Tea Blend

Let the gentle power of a chamomile tea blend transport you to a state of tranquility by calming your mind and soothing your spirit, thereby easing stress and promoting restful sleep.

**Ingredients:**

- 1 tbsp dried chamomile flowers
- 1 tsp dried mint leaves (optional)
- 1 tsp dried lavender flowers (optional)
- Honey or lemon (optional)

**Instructions:**

1. Boil fresh, filtered water and let it cool slightly.
2. Place the chamomile, mint, and lavender in a cup.
3. Pour the hot water over the herbs and cover.
4. Steep for 5–10 minutes.
5. Strain the mixture and, if desired, sweeten with honey or lemon.
6. Enjoy slowly, focusing on the calming aromas.

**Contraindications:**

- Those allergic to ragweed or related plants should use caution.

## Lavender Sleep Spray

Let the soothing aroma of a lavender sleep spray create a tranquil atmosphere, calming your mind and gently inviting sleep.

### Ingredients:

- 1 cup distilled water
- 10–15 drops lavender essential oil

### Instructions:

1. In a spray bottle, combine the distilled water and lavender essential oil.
2. Shake well before each use.
3. Lightly spritz over your pillow and bedding before sleeping.

### Contraindications:

- Generally safe; avoid if you have a known sensitivity to essential oils.

## Sage Smudging Ceremony

Let the ritual of smudging sage cleanse your space and uplift your spirit, inviting positive energy, purification, and mental clarity with every mindful movement.

### Ingredients:

- 1 dried sage bundle (ethically sourced)

### Instructions:

1. Gather your sage bundle.

2. Light the tip of the bundle until it begins to smolder and produce smoke.
3. Gently fan the smoke around the room or over yourself while focusing on your intention (e.g., clearing negativity).
4. Once finished, extinguish the bundle and store it safely for future use.

**Contraindications:**

- Avoid prolonged direct inhalation of smoke; use with caution if you are sensitive to smoke or have respiratory issues.

### Lemon Balm Tea

Let the refreshing blend of lemon balm tea brighten your day, ease your mind, and gently relax you.

**Ingredients:**

- 1 tbsp dried lemon balm leaves
- 1 tsp dried chamomile flowers
- Honey (optional)

**Instructions:**

1. Boil water and let it cool slightly.
2. Add the lemon balm and chamomile to a cup.
3. Pour the hot water over the herbs and steep for 5–7 minutes.
4. Strain the tea and sweeten it with honey if desired.

**Contraindications:**

- Generally safe; consult a healthcare professional if you are pregnant or have known allergies.

### Valerian Root Tea

Let the earthy strength of valerian root tea ease your mind and prepare you for a rejuvenating night by promoting relaxation and restorative sleep.

**Ingredients:**

- 1 tsp dried valerian root
- 1 cup boiling water
- 1 tsp honey (optional)
- Lemon (optional)

**Instructions:**

1. Boil water and let it cool slightly.
2. Place the valerian root in a cup and pour the hot water over it.
3. Steep for 10–15 minutes.
4. Strain and add honey or lemon if preferred.

**Contraindications:**

- May cause drowsiness; avoid operating heavy machinery after use.
- Not recommended for pregnant or breastfeeding women without professional guidance.

## Passionflower Tincture

Let the subtle power of passionflower tincture gently soothe your nerves with each measured drop for relaxation and anxiety relief.

### Ingredients:

- 1 part dried passionflower
- 1 part vodka or apple cider vinegar

### Instructions:

1. Combine the dried passionflower with your chosen liquid in a jar.
2. Seal the jar and shake well.
3. Store in a dark place for 4–6 weeks, shaking occasionally.
4. Strain the mixture and use a few drops as needed for anxiety relief.

### Contraindications:

- Consult with a healthcare provider before use if pregnant, breastfeeding, or taking prescription medications.

## Calming Essential Oil Blend

Let a blend of essential oils envelop you in soothing aromas, restoring balance and tranquility with every application to boost your mood and relieve stress.

### Ingredients:

- 5 drops lavender essential oil

- 5 drops bergamot essential oil
- 5 drops frankincense essential oil

**Instructions:**

1. Mix the essential oils in a small bottle.
2. Dilute with a carrier oil if applying directly to the skin.
3. Use in a diffuser or apply to pulse points for a calming effect.

**Contraindications:**

- Avoid using undiluted essential oils on the skin; consult a healthcare professional if you are pregnant or sensitive to essential oils.

## Bringing It All Together

We've journeyed through time to see how herbs like chamomile, lavender, and sage have played a key role in mental and spiritual well-being. These plants, cherished by ancient cultures, continue to offer natural alternatives for relaxation and purification.

Chamomile soothes anxiety and aids sleep with its calming bioactive compounds. Lavender's scent fights insomnia while sage purifies spaces and supports emotional balance. It's fascinating how these humble plants manage to connect the dots between our physical health and mental peace, echoing practices that aim to strengthen our bond with nature.

Our exploration doesn't end here; this is an invitation to incorporate the wisdom of herbs into your daily life. Whether you're sipping chamomile tea at bedtime, enjoying the calming aroma of lavender in your room, or engaging in a sage smudging ritual, these practices foster moments of tranquility in our hectic lives.

Embracing these age-old traditions can transform your routine activities into meaningful rituals, offering a reminder of the harmony between the human spirit and the natural world. So, take a deep breath, let these herbs weave their magic, and allow yourself to enjoy the peace they bring.

# Chapter 6: Women's Health and Herbal Remedies

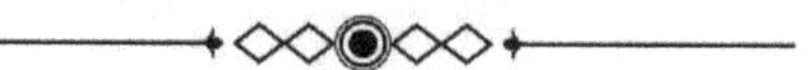

Exploring the vast world of women's health reveals a fascinating relationship between age-old herbal remedies and modern wellness practices. Herbal medicine has been an integral part of various cultures, serving as a natural approach to addressing women's health issues long before the advent of synthetic drugs.

This chapter explores the ancient herbal practices that have stood the test of time, highlighting their continued relevance in today's health-conscious society. By revisiting these botanical traditions, readers can uncover how nature's pharmacy has supported female well-being throughout history, offering insights into alternative ways of nurturing one's health holistically.

In this chapter, we'll set off on a journey through the healing properties and historical significance of certain herbs, notably raspberry leaf, fenugreek, and blue cohosh. These plants have been treasured for their unique benefits relating to menstrual health, fertility support, and childbirth assistance.

We will examine how raspberry leaf tea has been celebrated for menstrual comfort, delve into fenugreek's role as a fertility aid across civilizations, and uncover the trusted use of blue cohosh by midwives during childbirth. Each herb cited has its own story, complete with cultural roots and practical applications, connecting ancient wisdom with present-day practices. Throughout this exploration, we aim to deepen your understanding of how these herbal allies continue to support women's health in diverse and meaningful ways.

## Raspberry Leaf for Menstrual Health Support

Raspberry leaf has long been a staple in the realm of herbal remedies, particularly valued for addressing menstrual health. Historically, it's garnered recognition for its ability to regulate menstrual cycles and ease cramping.

Ancient herbalists greatly appreciated raspberry leaf for its uterine toning properties, which were believed to promote reproductive health by strengthening and relaxing the muscles in the pelvic area. These qualities made it an essential ally in women's health, especially since synthetic drugs weren't available at the time. Women would typically consume raspberry leaf as a tea, a gentle yet effective method to harness its benefits.

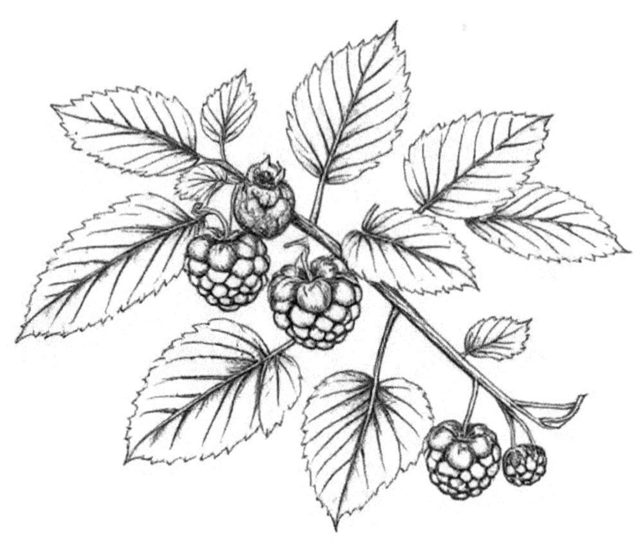

Rich in essential vitamins and minerals, raspberry leaf boasts high levels of vitamin C and magnesium, both crucial for hormone regulation. Vitamin C helps boost immunity and manage stress responses, which can be particularly beneficial during menstruation. Meanwhile, magnesium plays a pivotal role in muscle relaxation, reducing cramps and easing tension throughout the body. This nutrient composition supports overall reproductive health, making raspberry leaf a valuable addition to any woman's wellness routine.

In modern times, scientific research has begun to validate the traditional use of raspberry leaf. Studies indicate that its potential in treating menstrual discomfort is not mere folklore but grounded in reality. While more data is needed to fully understand its mechanisms, the convergence of ancient practices with contemporary science adds credibility to raspberry leaf's efficacy. For instance, the compound fragarine found in raspberry leaf is noted for its toning and tightening effect on uterine muscles, aligning with what herbalists have long advocated (Socha et al., 2023).

One doesn't need advanced herbal knowledge to benefit from raspberry leaf; it's quite easy to prepare. Typically consumed as a tea, this preparation provides a straightforward way to incorporate the herb into daily life. To make raspberry leaf tea, bring water to a boil, let it cool slightly, and then add two tbsp of dried raspberry leaves. Cover and steep for 15–30 minutes before straining. Sweeten to taste if desired. It's advised to source raspberry leaves ethically, ensuring they're organic and free from harmful pesticides—taking care that the product consists entirely of the leaves rather than stems or fillers enhances therapeutic impact (Torrens, 2022).

Beyond individual preparations, raspberry leaf is often found in tea blends that pair it with other herbs like peppermint or chamomile, enhancing flavor while complementing its medicinal virtues. These blends soothe, support hormonal balance, and alleviate menstrual discomfort. The mild diuretic effect of raspberry leaf further reduces water retention, a common issue during periods.

For many women around the world, raspberry leaf tea remains a trustworthy companion through various phases of life, from the challenges of adolescence to menopause. It provides comfort and relief, rooted in centuries of use, and it's steadily gaining recognition in the wellness community. While it is considered safe for most healthy adults, it's always best to consult with healthcare professionals, particularly during pregnancy, due to mixed evidence regarding its safety during early pregnancy stages (Torrens, 2022).

## Fenugreek in Ancient Fertility Aids

Fenugreek has long been celebrated as a fertility aid, a testament to its deep-rooted significance in various cultures worldwide. Across different civilizations, fenugreek has played a vital role in fertility rituals and traditions, symbolizing abundance and prosperity. In ancient Egypt, for example, it was believed that fenugreek could increase fertility, with women consuming it to improve their reproductive health and enhance the chances of conception. Similarly, in traditional Chinese medicine, fenugreek was utilized as a tonic to support female health and vitality.

The belief in fenugreek's ability to balance hormones is central to its use as a fertility enhancer. Fenugreek seeds are thought to influence estrogen production, which can positively impact menstrual cycle regulation. By supporting hormonal balance, fenugreek may contribute to more regular and less painful menstrual cycles, potentially aiding those who struggle with irregularities or discomfort. While scientific evidence remains limited, many users and practitioners of traditional medicine continue to advocate for fenugreek's potential benefits, pointing to centuries of anecdotal success stories.

A practical advantage of fenugreek lies in its versatility in culinary applications, offering an array of possibilities for those looking to incorporate it into their diet. One popular method involves creating fenugreek-infused oils, which can serve both culinary and therapeutic purposes. To make this oil at home, gently heat a base oil like olive or coconut oil and add fenugreek seeds, allowing them to infuse over low heat for about 20 minutes. This infusion can be used as a massage oil, which is reputed to support circulation and overall well-being. Additionally, incorporating fenugreek into food recipes is simple and rewarding. Fenugreek seeds, with their maple-like flavor, can be ground into powders and added to dishes such as curries or stews, enhancing both taste and potential health benefits.

In modern times, fenugreek continues to be relevant in the realm of fertility treatments and its usage persists among those seeking natural options. Although scientific studies remain scarce, numerous contemporary users report positive experiences with fenugreek in boosting fertility and libido. These personal accounts often highlight the herb's longstanding reputation and emphasize the need for more comprehensive research to better understand its effects.

## Midwives' Use of Blue Cohosh During Childbirth

Blue cohosh, a notable herb in women's health, has been used traditionally by midwives to support childbirth. Across generations, this herb has demonstrated its value in labor assistance thanks to the expertise and practices grounded in ancient childbirth support systems.

Midwives, who have long relied on natural remedies to aid in delivery, held blue cohosh in high regard for its purported ability to encourage uterine contractions, thereby facilitating smoother labors. The depth of their knowledge can be seen in the systematic incorporation of such herbal remedies into birthing practices, showcasing an intrinsic understanding of maternal health requirements and natural interventions.

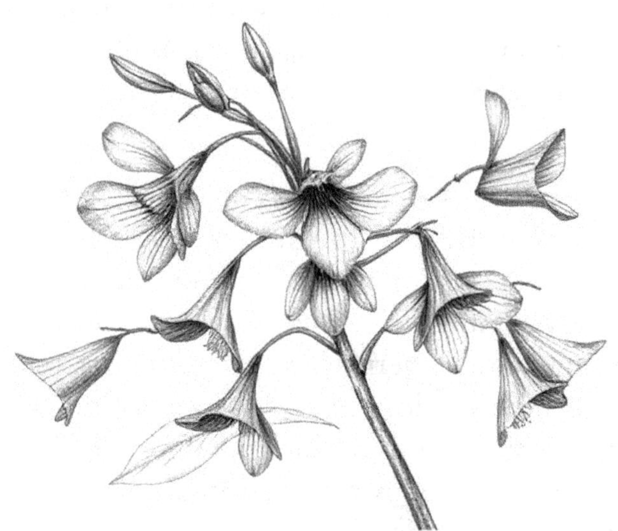

The mechanism by which blue cohosh operates lies in its unique compounds, which are believed to stimulate uterine contractions. This action is particularly valued during childbirth when enhancing contraction efficacy can lead to more straightforward labor experiences.

Old texts and oral traditions emphasize how these compounds have been utilized to manage labor more effectively, mitigating prolonged birth processes that could pose risks to both mother and child. The active components in blue cohosh include alkaloids and saponins, substances known for their potential physiological effects on the human body. It's essential to note that while these properties highlight the plant's traditional use as a labor aid, they also point to the necessity of informed application under professional guidance.

Culturally, blue cohosh holds significant importance in various childbirth rituals. It is often woven into the ceremonial fabric of different communities, symbolizing not just a practical tool but a spiritual one that enriches reproductive traditions. In many societies, this herb is considered a gift from nature to aid women in one of life's most transformative journeys. Its involvement in rituals underscores its perceived potency and reverence within cultures that prioritize holistic approaches to health and well-being. These cultural integrations serve to preserve heritage while promoting continuity in practice, illustrating how deeply rooted blue cohosh is within the narratives of childbirth across time and geography.

Despite its traditional significance, using blue cohosh requires careful consideration due to safety concerns. While it promises beneficial effects, there are critical guidelines that every prospective user must heed. First and foremost, consulting with experienced herbalists or healthcare providers familiar with herb-based medicine is crucial. Such experts can offer insights into appropriate usage, dosage, and potential interactions with other treatments or conditions.

Misuse or unsupervised consumption of blue cohosh has been linked to adverse effects, including neonatal complications as noted in historical case studies (McFarlin et al., 1999). Therefore, emphasizing collaboration with knowledgeable practitioners ensures that its application supports rather than compromises maternal and infant health.

Furthermore, McFarlin et al. (1999) provide further context for the deployment of herbs like blue cohosh in modern midwifery. Their study revealed that a considerable number of certified nurse-midwives incorporate herbal preparations, including blue cohosh, in labor stimulation protocols. The findings indicate a preference for natural methods over synthetic alternatives among certain practitioner groups, driven by an acknowledgment of traditional insights coupled with contemporary research validation.

However, the survey also highlights the cautionary stance of some practitioners who refrain from using such herbs due to insufficient empirical data on safety. This division underlines the need for a balanced approach that respects historical practices while demanding rigorous scientific scrutiny.

## Sacred Motherhood Recipes: Timeless Herbal Formulations for Fertility and Childbirth

Drawing on ancient wisdom, these recipes offer practical ways to incorporate traditional herbs into daily practices for supporting reproductive well-being and gentle childbirth. Presented below are clear, step-by-step guides to harness the natural benefits of fenugreek, blue cohosh, and raspberry leaf.

### Simple Recipes for a Special Time

Whether you're preparing for childbirth or supporting your body during a special time, these simple, natural recipes offer gentle ways to nurture your reproductive well-being with the wisdom of traditional herbs.

### Fenugreek Powder Seasoning

Let the warm, maple-like flavor of fenugreek enhance your dishes while contributing to potential fertility-related health benefits.

**Ingredients:**

- 1 cup fenugreek seeds

**Instructions:**

1. Roast the fenugreek seeds lightly in a dry skillet over low heat for 3–5 minutes until aromatic.
2. Allow the seeds to cool completely and then grind them into a fine powder using a spice grinder or mortar and pestle.

Use the fenugreek powder as a seasoning in curries, stews, or sprinkled over vegetables.

**Contraindications:**

- Those with a known allergy to fenugreek should avoid this remedy.
- Pregnant women should consult a healthcare provider before use, as fenugreek may influence hormonal activity.

## Blue Cohosh Tincture

Let the potent power of blue cohosh tincture serve as a natural aid to encourage uterine contractions to support labor—always use it under strict professional supervision.

**Ingredients:**

- 1 part dried blue cohosh root
- 1 part high-proof alcohol (such as vodka)

**Instructions:**

1. Place the dried blue cohosh root in a clean jar, filling it about halfway.
2. Pour enough high-proof alcohol over the herb to fully submerge it.
3. Seal the jar tightly and store it in a cool, dark place, shaking gently every day for 3–4 weeks.
4. Strain the infusion through a fine mesh or cheesecloth and transfer the liquid into a dark glass bottle for storage.

**Usage:** Only use this tincture under the guidance of a qualified healthcare professional.

**Contraindications:**

- Blue cohosh should never be used without expert supervision due to its potent effects and potential neonatal risks.
- Women with high-risk pregnancies or pre-existing health conditions should avoid it.

### Raspberry Leaf Tea

Let the soothing infusion of raspberry leaf tea ease menstrual discomfort and support fertility and reproductive well-being naturally.

**Ingredients:**

- 1 tbsp dried raspberry leaves
- 1 cup boiling water

**Instructions:**

1. Place the dried raspberry leaves in a teapot or heatproof cup.
2. Pour boiling water over the leaves and cover the container.
3. Allow the tea to steep for 10 minutes and then strain it into a cup.
4. Sip the tea slowly, enjoying its naturally earthy flavor and gentle benefits.

**Contraindications:**

- Raspberry leaf tea is generally safe; however, those with known allergies to the Rosaceae family of plants should use caution.
- Women who have specific medical conditions or are pregnant should consult a healthcare provider before regular use.

## Bringing It All Together

Throughout this chapter, we delved into the fascinating world of ancient herbal practices that have supported women's health for centuries. Starting with raspberry leaf, we've seen how it was used to ease menstrual discomfort and support reproductive well-being through its rich nutrient profile. Even today, its benefits are being explored by modern science, affirming its role in herbal medicine.

Meanwhile, fenugreek's reputation as a fertility enhancer demonstrated how herbs have been part of cultural beliefs and practices globally, offering potential hormonal balancing benefits. Additionally, blue cohosh provided insight into traditional childbirth practices, highlighting the deep-rooted significance of such herbs in various communities.

As we wrap up our exploration of these botanical wonders, it's clear that ancient wisdom continues to resonate in today's wellness routines. The long-standing use of these herbs serves as a testament to their enduring appeal and potential benefits, backed by emerging scientific validation.

While incorporating them into daily life can be easy and straightforward, it's always best to approach their use with mindfulness and professional guidance. By understanding the historical and cultural contexts of these plants, we not only appreciate their contributions to women's health but also honor the traditions that have carried them through generations.

# Chapter 7: Rituals and Remedies – The Spiritual Side of Healing

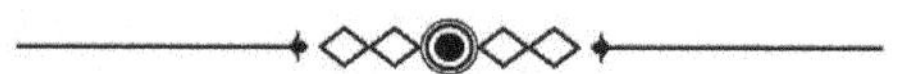

Rituals and remedies have always been a part of human societies, but when it comes to the spiritual side of healing, ancient cultures took it to another level. For them, spirituality and herbal practices weren't just complementary; they were interconnected in fascinating ways. Think of herbs not just as plants but as active participants in spiritual ecosystems that provide both physical and spiritual healing. This chapter explores this unique blend of spirituality and herbal wisdom, offering a glimpse into practices that may seem foreign yet surprisingly familiar in their intent to heal and nurture.

Let's set on a journey through time, exploring how ancient cultures used herbs in their rituals. You'll discover how Native American practices, with their deep reverence for nature, blended spiritual ceremonies with herbal knowledge to create powerful cleansing rituals. Alongside, we'll peek into sacred temple gardens of ancient civilizations where every plant had a purpose beyond mere sustenance. Finally, we'll visit ancient Rome, where herbs like hyssop and rue played vital roles in purification ceremonies.

This exploration will not only highlight different cultural perspectives but also instill a deeper understanding of our shared past, helping you appreciate the timeless value placed on the natural world for spiritual and physical well-being.

## Use of Herbs in Native American Smudging Ceremonies

In Native American traditions, the use of herbs in spiritual practices plays a significant role in maintaining balance and harmony with the natural world. These herbs are not only tools for physical healing but also critical elements for spiritual cleansing and connection.

Cedar, first and foremost, is revered for its powerful purification and protective qualities. In many ceremonies, cedar is burned, releasing transformative smoke that is believed to cleanse both the spirit and the physical surroundings. This act of purification is crucial as it clears away negative energies and creates a sacred space for rituals and gatherings.

The distinctive crackling sound when cedar burns is said to call the spirits' attention, inviting them to be present during the ceremony. This auditory signal is an essential aspect of spiritual communication, acknowledging the presence of ancestors and seeking guidance from the spiritual realm. Cedar is often laid on the ground inside sweat lodges, providing an added layer of protection and enhancing the spiritual experience of participants. Its use connects individuals with their ancestors, fostering a deep-rooted sense of identity and cultural continuity.

Sage, another pivotal herb, is commonly used to dispel negative energies and invite positive ones. Smudging with sage involves burning the dried leaves and using the smoke to purify people, spaces, and objects. This ritual serves to cleanse the mind and body, preparing individuals for spiritual activities or important life transitions. By removing negativity, sage encourages mental wellness, allowing individuals to approach life with clarity and peace.

This practice highlights the intricate link between spirituality and mental health, highlighting how traditional methods provide a holistic approach to well-being. Sage's potent aroma is believed to have medicinal properties, reinforcing its role not just as a spiritual tool but as a means to promote physical health. In this way, sage embodies the interconnectedness of body, mind, and spirit, serving as a bridge between these facets of existence.

Sweetgrass, recognized for its sweet scent, symbolizes kindness and calls forth good spirits. When used in smudging ceremonies, sweetgrass releases a pleasant aroma that has a calming effect on participants. This herb is often used after sage, inviting beneficial energies that replace those dispelled by sage.

Sweetgrass braids—a popular form—are crafted by intertwining 21 strands, which are symbolic of the community and the connection between past, present, and future generations. The gentle nature of sweetgrass makes it a perfect symbol of Mother Earth's nurturing qualities, reminding practitioners of the importance of kindness and gratitude in their interactions with others and the environment. It highlights the idea that spiritual practices are not isolated rituals but integral parts of daily life, encouraging ongoing positive interaction with the world.

Tobacco holds a unique place in Native American spirituality, symbolizing respect and gratitude. It is often offered as a gift to elders, healers, and the Creator, acknowledging the wisdom and guidance they provide. Tobacco is considered the primary plant among sacred medicines and is central to many ceremonies and offerings.

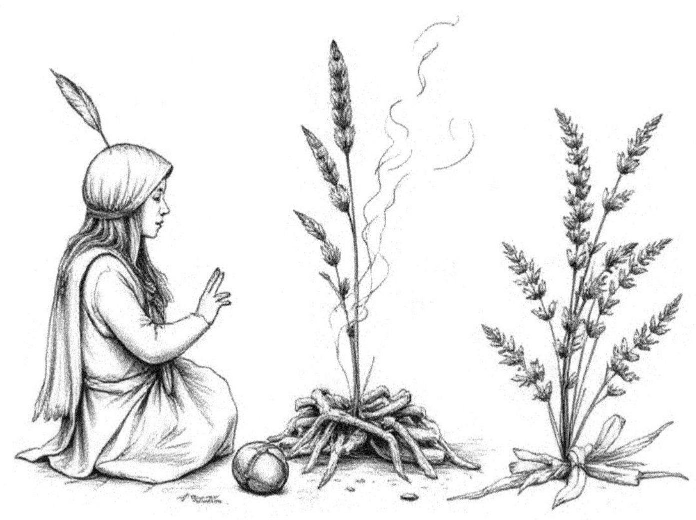

The act of offering tobacco is seen as a way to communicate prayers and intentions to the spiritual world, facilitating a deeper connection with the ancestors.

This practice emphasizes the value placed on relationships within the community and with the spiritual realm. The traditional use of tobacco differs significantly from its commercial consumption, focusing on its sacred role rather than its addictive properties. It acts as a mediator in spiritual dialogue, ensuring that messages and requests are heard and acknowledged by the divine entities.

These herbal practices collectively underscore the profound link between herbs and spirituality in Native American cultures. They reflect a worldview where plants are not mere resources but active participants in the spiritual ecosystem. Each herb serves a specific role, whether it is purifying, protecting, or inviting positive energies.

More than just tools, herbs are viewed as living beings with whom humans must maintain a respectful relationship. Ritualistic use fosters community bonds and spiritual awareness, creating a shared understanding of their cultural and spiritual significance. This interaction illustrates the sophisticated knowledge and respect indigenous communities hold for the natural world.

## Sacred Herbal Gardens in Ancient Temples

In ancient cultures, sacred spaces for cultivating herbs played a crucial role in both spiritual and communal practices. These temple gardens were not just plots of land; they represented an intertwining of the physical and spiritual realms, essential for the holistic well-being of their communities. Through these sacred spaces, we can gather valuable insights into the reverence for nature that characterized many ancient societies.

Temple gardens served as dedicated spaces where healing herbs were grown with great care and respect. These gardens were often part of religious or communal sanctuaries, emphasizing the deep connection between nature and spirituality. The presence of these gardens symbolized a commitment to health, healing, and spiritual growth.

These gardens were not just about maintaining physical well-being but also nurturing spiritual health, as they served as sources of remedies for spiritual and physical ailments. By offering easy access to a wide array of medicinal herbs, temple gardens played a vital role in daily spiritual life, reminding individuals of their responsibilities toward both nature and their community.

The gardens were more than mere sources of medicine; they were considered living libraries of herbal knowledge. This knowledge was diligently carried forward through generations, often transmitted orally or through hands-on learning. Such transmission highlighted the importance of these gardens as repositories of wisdom, ensuring that the knowledge did not die with any single generation but continued to benefit the community for generations to come.

The teachings from these gardens often included understanding the properties of various plants, how to harvest them sustainably, and how to prepare effective remedies. This practice of passing down knowledge fostered a sense of continuity and respect for tradition, ensuring that people remained connected to their history and culture.

Rituals also played a significant role in these sacred spaces, with specific ceremonies designed to honor the spirits of the herbs themselves. Honoring plant spirits was an integral part of blending spiritual practice with herbalism. For instance, rituals might involve offerings or prayers to the deity or spirit associated with a particular plant before harvesting it.

Such practices acknowledged the perceived sentient nature of the plants and showed gratitude for their healing powers. Rituals often served dual purposes: enhancing the efficacy of the herbal remedies and reinforcing communal bonds. By gathering for these rituals, communities could celebrate their shared beliefs and strengthen their social structures.

These practices reflect a broader cultural attitude that values interconnectedness between humans and nature. Respecting the natural world meant acknowledging its role in spiritual and physical well-being and acting as stewards of its delicate balance. This reverence for nature teaches modern generations the importance of sustainable practices and respect for the environment.

The cultivation and use of temple gardens illustrate a model of sustainability and community engagement that resonates even today. As contemporary society grapples with environmental challenges, lessons from these ancient practices remind us of the value of working harmoniously with nature. The historical perspective on sacred gardens encourages us to consider how modern gardening and herbal practices might incorporate similar principles of respect, responsibility, and reverence for the natural world.

## Role of Herbs in Roman Purification Rituals

In ancient Rome, the integration of herbs into spiritual rituals was more than a practice; it was an essential aspect of their cultural and religious identity. Herbs like hyssop and rue were vital in various purification ceremonies, which reflected a significant spiritual emphasis on cleanliness.

Hyssop, often known as the "holy herb," was revered for its purifying qualities and used extensively to cleanse both people and spaces (*Hyssop (Niu Xi Cao)*, 2023). The application of hyssop in purification rites highlighted the Romans' belief that physical cleanliness facilitated spiritual purity. Rue, another herb commonly employed, was known for its protective properties, warding off evil influences and ensuring spiritual safety.

The utilization of these herbs was not limited to personal rituals; they played crucial roles in both military and public rites. During significant events, such as military campaigns or public celebrations, specific herbal sacrifices were performed. These practices were not only symbolic but also pragmatic, aimed at securing divine favor for communal well-being. Soldiers would carry sprigs of these potent herbs as talismans, believing they offered protection and courage on the battlefield. This tradition underscored how deeply ingrained herbal practices were in Roman society, blending practical applications with spiritual significance.

Furthermore, the commercial distribution and trade of these herbal remedies facilitated the spread of purification rituals across the vast empire. Markets became hubs where various herbs could be accessed by those from different regions, enhancing both local and widespread knowledge and use. This trade network ensured that the benefits of these herbs were not confined to the urban elite but reached rural communities as well, supporting a shared cultural heritage centered around spiritual health and protection. The widespread availability of these herbs enabled many to engage in rituals that might have been otherwise inaccessible due to geographic or economic barriers.

The symbolic representation of herbs in Roman art and literature further emphasized their importance. For instance, laurel and verbena were depicted in various artworks, each embodying virtues such as protection and invincibility. These depictions were not mere artistic expressions but served as powerful reminders of the inherent strength and sanctity attributed to these plants. As such, they reinforced the societal value placed on herbal practices and their perceived influence on daily life and spiritual well-being. This symbolism continued to shape modern practices, preserving the legacy of ancient traditions.

The rich tradition of integrating herbs into spiritual practices demonstrates the broader cultural significance of herbs in Roman society. The deliberate selection and ceremonial use of herbs like hyssop and rue illustrate a deep-rooted appreciation for the natural world and its capacity to support human spirituality and community cohesion. By examining these practices, we gain valuable insights into how ancient civilizations viewed the intersection of the spiritual and natural realms, enriching our understanding of historical approaches to holistic health and wellness.

## Celestial Herbal Ceremonies: Timeless Rituals for Spiritual Renewal

These rituals blend ancient herbal wisdom with spiritual practice, offering a mindful pathway to cleanse, protect, and nurture your inner self. Each ceremony is presented with a brief description, followed by clear instructions so you can easily integrate these time-honored practices into your modern routine.

### Simple Rituals You Can Follow

These easy-to-follow rituals are designed to bring balance and mindfulness into your daily routine, helping you connect with your body and spirit.

## Cedar Smudging Ritual

Let the ancient power of cedar purify and protect your space and provide access to ancestral wisdom.

**Ingredients:**

- Dried cedar bundle or cedar sticks

**Instructions:**

1. Light the tip of the cedar bundle until it begins to smolder and produce fragrant smoke.
2. Gently fan the smoke around your body and throughout the room, focusing on clearing away negativity and inviting positivity.
3. Continue until the space feels cleansed and refreshed.

**Contraindications:**

- Avoid prolonged direct inhalation of smoke. Use with caution if you are sensitive to smoke or have respiratory issues.

## Sage Smudging Ritual

Let the sacred smoke of sage purify your surroundings and mind of negative energies and invite positive forces.

**Ingredients:**

- Dried sage bundle

**Instructions:**

1. Light the sage bundle and allow it to smolder until it produces ample smoke.

2. Use your hand or a feather to gently direct the smoke over your body and throughout the space, setting your intentions for purification and renewal.
3. Allow the smoke to linger before gently extinguishing the bundle.

**Contraindications:**

- Use caution if you have respiratory sensitivities. Avoid prolonged exposure.

### Sweetgrass Offering Ritual

Let the uplifting aroma of sweetgrass create an atmosphere of kindness and gratitude by inviting benevolent spirits and nurturing community harmony.

**Ingredients:**

- Sweetgrass braid (traditionally braided with 21 strands)

**Instructions:**

1. After completing your smudging ceremony, gently wave the sweetgrass braid around your space or over yourself.
2. As you do so, recite a brief prayer or affirmation to invite positive energy and reinforce community bonds.

**Contraindications:**

- Generally safe; ensure you are not allergic to sweetgrass.

## Tobacco Offering Ritual

Let the ritual use of traditional tobacco serve as a respectful mediator between the physical and spiritual realms, honoring ancestors and establishing a sacred connection.

**Ingredients:**

- Traditional Native American tobacco (natural, unprocessed)

**Instructions:**

- Light a small amount of tobacco in a fireproof bowl. Hold the bowl respectfully and allow the smoke to rise as you silently offer your prayers and intentions to the spiritual realm.

**Contraindications:**

- Use only as a sacred offering. Avoid recreational inhalation or excessive use.

## Roman Purification Ritual

Let the ancient methods of Roman purification inspire your own ritual using hyssop and rue to cleanse spaces and invite divine favor.

**Ingredients:**

- Sprigs of hyssop
- Sprigs of rue

**Instructions:**

- Light a small bundle of hyssop until it gently smolders, releasing purifying smoke.
- Pass the sprigs of rue through the hyssop smoke and then wave them around the room in sweeping motions to cleanse and protect the area.
- Optionally, recite a brief invocation or prayer to set your intention for purification.

**Contraindications:**

- Use for ritual purposes only. Avoid ingestion and exercise caution if you have sensitivities.

## Temple Garden Blessing Ritual

- Let this ritual connect you with the nurturing energy of nature's bounty to honor the sacred herbal garden and invoke spiritual growth.

**Ingredients:**

- A selection of fresh herbs from your garden (such as basil, rosemary, or thyme)

**Instructions:**

1. Gather a small assortment of fresh herbs from your garden and arrange them in a decorative bowl as an offering.
2. Light a candle nearby and, with reverence, speak a blessing or prayer for the garden and its gifts.
3. Allow the herbs to remain as a symbol of your ongoing connection to nature.

**Contraindications:**

- None; simply ensure the herbs are organically grown and fresh.

## Bringing It All Together

The chapter delved into how ancient cultures uniquely intertwined spirituality with herbal practices. We explored Native American ceremonies, where cedar, sage, sweetgrass, and tobacco each played important roles in spiritual rituals. These herbs were far more than just healing tools; they helped cleanse the spirit, create sacred spaces, and connect individuals to their ancestors.

Through smudging ceremonies and offerings, these practices highlighted a deep respect for the natural world and its impact on both mental and physical well-being. The exploration of temple gardens from other ancient societies revealed similar themes, emphasizing the importance of sustainable interactions between humans and nature.

We also learned about the Romans' use of herbs like hyssop and rue in purification rituals. These powerful plants were integral to personal, military, and public ceremonies, demonstrating their cultural significance. The trade and depiction of herbs throughout the Roman Empire further underscored their importance in everyday life.

By examining these practices across different cultures, we're reminded of the enduring connection between spirituality and the natural world. It shows us how ancient wisdom can still offer valuable insights into our modern quest for holistic health and mindfulness, encouraging us to reconnect with nature in meaningful ways.

# Chapter 8: Building Your Own Herbarium

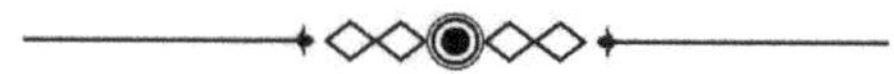

Creating your own herbarium is like building a personal wellness arsenal right in the comfort of your home. You surround yourself with the tools and knowledge to harness the power of herbs, tailored to meet your health needs. Imagine having the perfect blend of natural remedies at your fingertips, waiting to be transformed into soothing teas, invigorating tinctures, or aromatic balms. The allure here is in crafting something deeply personal and functional—a space that reflects your holistic journey while being incredibly practical and beneficial for everyday life.

In this chapter, we're diving into the essentials of setting up a thriving herbarium from scratch. Understanding proper herb storage is crucial, as it ensures your collection remains potent and effective over time. We'll explore how to choose the best containers and storage environments to keep your herbs at their best.

Furthermore, you'll learn about must-have tools that simplify the process of preparing your herbs, ensuring you get the most out of each one. From grinding with a mortar and pestle to accurate measuring, these elements are foundational to any herbal enthusiast's toolkit. We'll also cover tips on growing your own herbs, even if you're short on space.

Whether it's container gardening or finding the right spots in your home, creating a mini garden is simpler than you might think. By the end of this chapter, you'll have a comprehensive guide to not only store and utilize your herbs effectively but also cultivate them, bringing your herbarium dreams to life.

## Proper Herb Storage

Storing herbs properly is critical in maintaining their potency and effectiveness. If you're building your home herbarium, you need to ensure that the therapeutic properties of these natural treasures are preserved for as long as possible. The first step toward this is understanding the optimal conditions for herb storage: cool, dark, and dry places.

Why is this important? It's because heat, light, and moisture are the enemies of dried herbs. They can accelerate degradation, leading to a loss of flavor, aroma, and therapeutic value. Storing herbs in an environment that minimizes these factors helps retain their natural oils and active compounds, which are responsible for their healing properties.

A practical guideline to follow is choosing a location like a pantry or a cupboard away from direct sunlight or any heat sources like ovens and stoves. Avoid storing them in high-humidity areas such as above sinks or near bathroom windows. By keeping your herbs in the right environment, you'll be maximizing their shelf life and ensuring that they remain potent and effective when you need them.

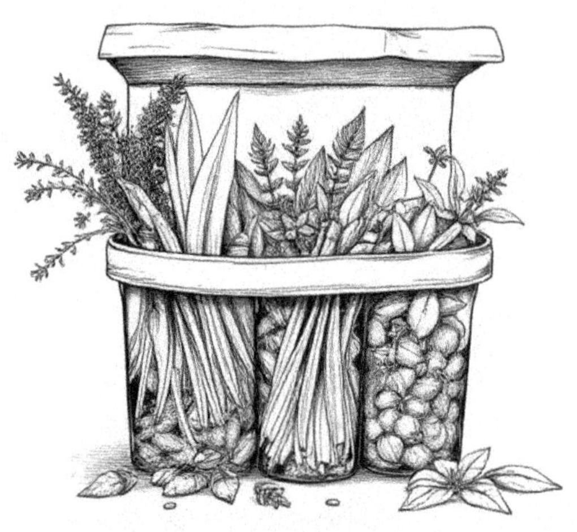

Next, let's talk about the containers. Glass jars are often recommended for storing herbs because they offer significant protection against air and light exposure, which are detrimental to the quality of herbs. Unlike plastic, glass doesn't leach chemicals, ensuring that what you've stored maintains its purity.

Mason jars with good sealing lids, or specialized dark-tinted glass jars, are ideal choices. They block out light and prevent air from entering, thereby preserving the freshness of your herbs. For additional protection, choose opaque or tinted jars if space allows. They work exceptionally well if you can't store herbs in a completely dark area since they cut down light exposure considerably.

Understanding the varying shelf lives of different herbs also plays a crucial role in planning their usage and maintaining your supply. While some herbs, like bay leaves, can last up to two years when stored correctly, others like basil and chives may only maintain peak potency for about a year. A helpful tip here is to label your jars with the date of storage. This simple practice aids in easily tracking freshness and ensures you're using herbs at their best. It's also wise to prioritize using herbs with shorter shelf lives first to make sure nothing goes to waste.

Speaking of reducing waste, implementing a rotation system is a smart strategy for managing your inventory. Similar to how supermarkets handle stock, you should place newly harvested or purchased herbs at the back, moving older ones to the front. This encourages you to use them before their potency fades. Think of it like managing a library; cycling through the collection keeps everything fresh and in top condition. This system not only preserves efficacy but also saves money by reducing unnecessary purchases and minimizing spoilage.

Another fun way to keep track of rotation is by having a checklist or chart where you periodically review each jar's contents. This gives you a snapshot of your current inventory and acts as a gentle reminder to use what you have before it loses its potency.

Additionally, think about how much of each herb you actually use regularly. Buying or harvesting in small quantities more frequently is another effective way to ensure you always have fresh herbs on hand. It's tempting to stock up but remember that the fresher the herb, the more robust its effects will be.

Establishing a routine for checking your herbs is beneficial too. Perhaps every few months, set aside a day to inspect your collection. Look for signs that herbs have passed their prime—discoloration, lack of scent, or obvious moisture content. Doing so not only keeps your apothecary organized but also allows you to determine which herbs have been most useful and which might need replenishing or replacing.

Combining these practices into your routine preserves each herb's potency, lengthens its usability, and enhances the overall satisfaction and efficacy of your herbal craft. Proper storage is a fundamental aspect of building a thriving home herbarium that serves your health and wellness needs effectively. Remember, it's not just about having a variety of herbs; it's about maintaining their quality to harness the full potential of nature's remedies.

## Must-Have Tools for Herbal Preparation

When setting up your herbarium, the right tools can truly make all the difference. Let's start with the classic mortar and pestle. This humble tool is a must-have for anyone serious about herbal preparation. It might seem old-fashioned, but its role in an herbarium cannot be overstated.

## Mortar and Pestle

By manually grinding herbs with a mortar and pestle, you can preserve their active components much better than electronic grinders would. This is especially important when you're using herbs for both culinary and medicinal purposes, as these active components are often what provide the desired effects.

To use a mortar and pestle effectively, you need to understand the correct way to grind different textures of herbs. Some require firm pressure; others demand a gentle touch. Start by placing small amounts of the herb into the mortar. Use the pestle to apply force in circular motions. This technique releases the oils and essence needed for potent results, whether you're brewing an herbal tea or concocting a soothing balm.

After you've ground your herbs, straining becomes an important step. This is where herbal strainers and cheesecloths come in handy. These tools ensure that your teas and tinctures come out clean and potent. It's essential to get this part right because any leftover plant material can affect the taste or effectiveness of your preparation.

## Strainer and Cheesecloth

Using a strainer is pretty straightforward. For liquids, like teas, simply pour through the strainer to catch any solid bits. A cheesecloth is excellent for other textures. If you're making tinctures or infused oils, line your strainer with cheesecloth to double-filter for a clearer result. Fold it in layers over the strainer and use it to squeeze every last drop from your mixture. Cleanliness is key here, so ensure your tools are washed and dried thoroughly after each use to prevent contamination.

## Measuring Tools

Next up, accurate measuring tools are vital in any herbarium. When dealing with herbal remedies, consistency is crucial. You want the dosage to be just right every time, and good measuring tools help achieve that. While it's tempting to eyeball quantities, investing in some precise scales and measuring spoons will do wonders for the accuracy of your preparations. Consistent measurements ensure that each batch you make has the same strength, allowing you to monitor and adjust dosages as needed for optimal health benefits.

Having a set of kitchen scales that measure even small quantities accurately is beneficial. Opt for scales that offer gram-level precision. They are especially useful when creating products like capsules or blends that require exact amounts of each ingredient. Additionally, consider acquiring graduated cylinders or droppers for liquid measures, which are perfect for preparing solutions or extracts.

## Glass Jars and Bottles

Moving on, let's talk about glass jars and bottles. These are not only for storage but also for preserving the quality of your herbs long-term. Unlike plastic containers, glass doesn't react with herbs, ensuring that there's no unwanted chemical interaction. This is particularly important for maintaining the herbs' potency and safety.

Storing your herbs in glass ensures that they remain free from contaminants and maintain their integrity. Consider using tinted glass containers if possible, as they can help reduce light exposure, which can degrade herbs over time. Furthermore, proper labeling is a must. Clearly mark each jar with contents and dates of storage, keeping everything organized and easy to access.

It's also worth noting that storage conditions matter. Although this will be discussed later, remember that where you store these jars can greatly affect the herbs' longevity. Even though we've covered essential tools, integrating them into a routine requires practice. Regular and mindful use of these tools will enhance your confidence in managing an herbarium at home.

## Growing Herbs in Small Spaces

A home herbarium brimming with fresh herbs sounds like a slice of herbal heaven, doesn't it? The good news is that you don't need acres of garden space to make this dream a reality. With a bit of creativity and some practical know-how, container gardening becomes your best friend in crafting your unique herbal haven.

Container gardening offers remarkable flexibility, allowing you to transform even the tiniest of spaces into a thriving herb oasis. Picture a sunny windowsill or a small balcony; these are the perfect spots to start your journey.

The power of container gardening lies in its adaptability. You can use pots, hanging baskets, or even repurpose old tin cans. Each container becomes a mini garden, where herbs can establish their cozy little homes. This approach not only saves space but also lets you move plants around to catch the sunlight as the seasons change.

Now, the success of your urban garden depends heavily on choosing the right herbs. While it might be tempting to pick every herb under the sun, consider starting with those that are comfortable in confined conditions. Herbs like basil, mint, and chives thrive in containers and handle low-light situations well. They add flavor to your meals and turn any corner they occupy into a fragrant delight. When selecting herbs, think about their growth habits and preferences. Some prefer full sun, while others are shade lovers. By matching the environment to the plant's needs, you'll set up each herb for a successful life in its container.

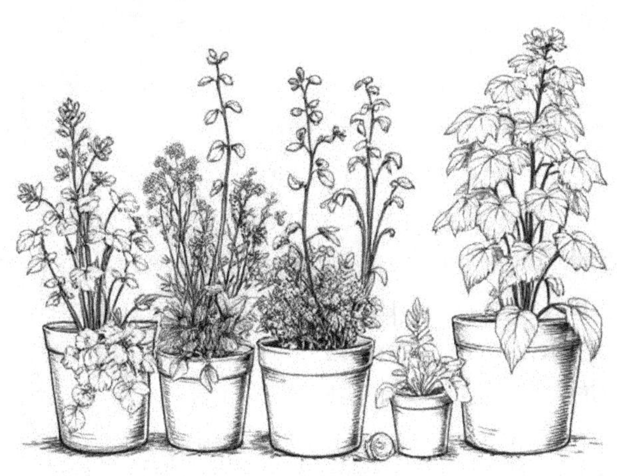

Once you've selected your herbs, the next step is ensuring they stay happy and healthy. Establishing a solid care routine is key. Watering is particularly crucial in containers because soil tends to dry out faster. Get into the habit of checking the soil moisture regularly. A simple touch test usually does the trick—if the top inch feels dry, it's time for a drink. But beware of overwatering, which can be just as problematic as underwatering. Adjust your watering schedule based on weather conditions and the specific needs of each herb.

Pest management is another aspect to keep an eye on. In a limited space, pests can quickly become a menace. Regularly inspect your herb leaves for any signs of trouble, such as yellowing or holes. If pests do invade, natural remedies like neem oil or a gentle soap spray can help keep them at bay without harming your precious plants.

Keeping your containers clean and free from dead leaves also helps prevent pest attraction.

As your herbs flourish, the exciting task of harvesting follows. Timing is everything here. Harvesting herbs at their peak ensures you capture the best flavor and potency. For leafy herbs like basil or mint, grow them until they have several sets of leaves, then pinch off the tops. This not only provides a flavorful addition to your culinary creations but also encourages bushier growth. With flowering herbs like lavender or chamomile, pick them just before they reach full bloom to retain their aromatic oils so they are in optimal condition for infusions or potpourris.

When you harvest strategically, you're not only enjoying a bountiful supply of herbs but also promoting continuous growth. Proper harvesting methods ensure that you're not stripping the plants bare, which would stress them excessively. Instead, by taking only what you need, you allow the plants to regenerate, providing a sustainable supply for future needs.

## Herbal Starter Kit: Essential Versatile Herbs for Multiple Remedies

1. **Chamomile:** A gentle herb prized for its calming and anti-inflammatory properties, ideal for soothing teas, herbal baths, and sleep aids.
2. **Lavender:** Renowned for its relaxing aroma and healing qualities, lavender is perfect for sleep

sprays, aromatherapy, and gentle topical applications.

3. **Sage:** Valued for its powerful purifying and cleansing properties, sage is useful in smudging ceremonies and herbal infusions for mental clarity.
4. **Lemon Balm:** A versatile herb that promotes relaxation and enhances mood; it's great for teas, tinctures, and digestive support.
5. **Rosemary:** A culinary staple that is also beneficial for memory and focus and as an ingredient in cleansing and revitalizing remedies.
6. **Mint:** Refreshing and soothing, mint is excellent for digestive teas and cooling infusions and as a natural remedy for minor digestive discomfort.
7. **Ginger:** Known for its warming and digestive properties, ginger is a key ingredient in teas that relieve nausea and support gut health.
8. **Turmeric:** Celebrated for its potent anti-inflammatory and antioxidant effects, it's widely used in golden milk, tinctures, and topical balms.
9. **Garlic:** A powerful antimicrobial and immune booster, garlic can be incorporated into infused oils, tinctures, and everyday cooking for health benefits.
10. **Raspberry Leaf:** Traditionally used for supporting reproductive health, raspberry leaf is excellent in teas and other gentle remedies that support women's well-being.

## Bringing It All Together

Creating a personalized herbarium at home is a delightful journey that blends tradition with practicality. This chapter has walked you through the essentials of herb storage, ensuring your collection remains potent and effective. By focusing on optimal storage conditions—cool, dark, and dry environments, you safeguard the therapeutic properties of your herbs. Choosing the right containers, like glass jars, helps maintain purity and prolongs shelf life.

We've also touched on practical strategies for managing inventory, such as labeling jars with storage dates and implementing a rotation system to maximize freshness and minimize waste. These steps are not just about preserving herbs; they're about enhancing their healing power and getting the most out of every leaf and root you use.

Equipped with this knowledge, you're now ready to build a thriving herb collection tailored to your needs. Whether you're storing bay leaves or nurturing basil in small spaces, understanding each herb's unique requirements ensures they stay fresh and effective. Establishing routines for checking and rotating your stash keeps everything organized and functional.

Remember, it's not just about collecting a variety of herbs; it's about nurturing their quality to harness the full potential of nature's remedies. Embrace these practices, and you'll find that your home herbarium soon becomes a source of wellness and satisfaction, providing natural solutions that enrich both body and spirit.

# Chapter 9: Modern Science Meets Ancient Wisdom

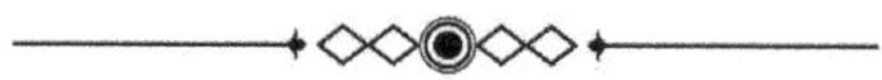

Integrating ancient herbal practices with modern scientific validation is like opening a treasure chest of time-tested remedies and mixing them with cutting-edge research. The idea of bringing together the best of both worlds can spark curiosity in even the most skeptical minds. Imagine discovering that the age-old remedies your grandparents swore by weren't just tales passed down for generations but forms of medicine with real, tangible benefits rooted in scientific evidence. It's like finding out that your grandma's recipe for chicken soup actually holds up under the microscope! This chapter looks into how turmeric, a seemingly simple spice, bridges the fascinating gap between old knowledge and new discoveries.

We'll explore how turmeric's anti-inflammatory properties, long hailed in traditional medicine systems, are gaining credibility through scientific research. You'll learn about curcumin, the powerhouse compound in turmeric that's capturing the medical community's attention.

While we will refer to recent studies that highlight turmeric's potential benefits for common inflammatory conditions like arthritis, we will also go beyond what today's science says, revisiting the historical backdrop of turmeric use across cultures, showing how these age-old applications are finding their place in modern kitchens and medicine cabinets.

Whether it's used in a comforting cup of golden milk or sprinkled over dishes, turmeric is a practical example of how ancient and modern wisdom come together to enhance well-being.

## Turmeric's Anti-Inflammatory Properties

In modern science, turmeric stands as a testament to how ancient wisdom can benefit from contemporary validation. Research has firmly established that curcumin, the active compound in turmeric, plays a significant role in reducing inflammation—a common thread linking it to modern medicinal practices and centuries-old remedies.

Recent clinical trials have highlighted curcumin's efficacy in mitigating inflammation markers, especially for conditions like osteoarthritis and rheumatoid arthritis. These chronic inflammatory disorders often lead to discomfort and diminished quality of life, prompting a demand for effective treatments with minimal side effects. Curcumin fits this bill perfectly.

For instance, in a systematic review involving several randomized controlled trials, curcumin was shown to alleviate symptoms associated with rheumatoid arthritis by modulating various inflammatory pathways (Kou et al., 2023). Patients reported decreased pain and swelling, which underscores curcumin's potential as an anti-inflammatory agent without the burden of serious side effects typically associated with conventional pharmaceuticals.

Moreover, historical references from India provide a vivid backdrop to turmeric's therapeutic applications. Ancient Ayurvedic texts document the use of turmeric as a remedy for injuries and chronic pain management, reflecting its deep-rooted place in traditional medicine systems.

These accounts are not fleeting mentions but robust endorsements repeatedly appearing across herbal manuals and practitioner anecdotes. Such historical usage is now gaining scientific backing, adding layers of credibility to these ancient practices. It's fascinating how today's scientists echo the sentiments of those who vouched for turmeric centuries ago.

Turmeric's multifaceted action lies in its ability to modulate inflammatory mediators and its impressive antioxidant properties. These characteristics offer an explanation for its effectiveness in reducing oxidative stress and inflammation, both factors playing pivotal roles in chronic disease progression. The mechanisms involve interfering with cellular signaling pathways that propagate inflammation and protect cells from oxidative damage. This dual approach not only addresses symptom reduction but also provides a protective shield against potential cellular deterioration over time (Daily et al., 2016).

When considering turmeric's practical applications, incorporating it into daily diets offers a simple yet powerful strategy for harnessing its benefits. One popular method is golden milk, a traditional Indian beverage combining turmeric with milk and sometimes other spices like ginger or cinnamon. Thanks to the fats and piperine found in some recipes, this preparation not only enhances the bioavailability of curcumin but also makes consuming a health supplement into a comforting ritual. Beyond beverages, turmeric can be seamlessly integrated into meals, such as curries, soups, or roasted vegetables.

However, understanding dosage and safe consumption is crucial to maximizing benefits while minimizing risks. Curcumin supplements often come in higher concentrations than what you'd typically find in dietary turmeric. Experts generally recommend consulting healthcare providers for personalized advice, especially since individual health conditions might dictate specific needs. It's also worth noting that excessive intake might not equate to increased benefits and could even pose health risks. Thus, moderation is key.

## Echinacea's Role in Immune Health

Echinacea is a fascinating example of how ancient herbal practices are being revisited through the lens of modern science. Historically, indigenous peoples across North America valued Echinacea for its impressive medicinal properties, using it extensively for wound healing and immune system support. This historical grounding is now buttressed by contemporary scientific research that paints a compelling picture of Echinacea's relevance today.

A critical aspect of modern Echinacea use revolves around its ability to prevent and treat common colds and flu. Recent studies have shown that Echinacea can reduce the duration of these illnesses, which is why it's become a popular choice in many households (*Echinacea*, 2024b). The idea here is quite simple: by taking Echinacea at the first sign of a cold, individuals may experience fewer symptoms and a quicker recovery. This aligns perfectly with traditional uses, where it was often applied as an all-round health booster.

Digging deeper, the understanding of Echinacea's benefits can be traced back to key constituents within the plant itself. Alkamides and polysaccharides are two primary compounds found in Echinacea, notably enhancing immune function. Scientific validation has demonstrated that these compounds interact with the immune system, thus underpinning Echinacea's historical reputation. Empirical evidence shows that these active components stimulate certain types of white blood cells, bolstering the body's defense mechanisms against pathogens (*Echinacea*, 2024a). This scientific backing not only gives credit to traditional methods but also emphasizes the potential of Echinacea in modern healthcare.

While acknowledging these scientific advancements, it's crucial to remember the authentic preparation methods used by indigenous communities. Their traditional knowledge surrounding Echinacea wasn't just about what parts of the plant to use but how they were prepared. For instance, early users of Echinacea would often prepare teas or apply topical pastes directly to wounds to leverage both internal and external healing properties. This hands-on approach laid a robust foundation for its medicinal significance, which contemporary practice continues to build upon.

When transitioning from history to practical application, it becomes necessary to explore the optimal ways to incorporate Echinacea into daily routines. Presently, consumers can choose from various forms like tinctures, teas, and capsules. These choices offer flexibility, tailoring usage to individual preferences and needs. For those new to Echinacea, starting with teas may provide a gentler introduction, while regular users might prefer the concentrated effects of a tincture. Capsules also present a convenient option, especially for those who travel and need easy access to their supplements.

However, one of the most important guidelines when using Echinacea—or any herbal supplement for that matter—is ensuring product quality. Different Echinacea products offer different levels of potency. High-quality Echinacea should have authentic labeling, detailing the species used and the part of the plant processed. Furthermore, sourcing transparent brands committed to sustainable and ethical production practices can make a substantial difference in efficacy and safety (*Echinacea*, 2024b).

Moreover, integrating such supplements into one's lifestyle requires one to be mindful of possible allergic reactions and interactions. While generally safe for short-term use, some people may experience mild effects like digestive discomfort. As with anything dietary, moderation is key, and consulting with a healthcare provider prior to use can provide additional reassurance.

## St. John's Wort for Depression Treatment

St. John's Wort, scientifically known as *Hypericum perforatum*, has gained popularity as a natural treatment for mild to moderate depression. Modern science has started to validate what ancient traditions have long held—that this herb can truly support emotional health. But let's delve deeper into how it works, its historical roots, and the necessary precautions one should take.

Clinical reviews have consistently highlighted the effectiveness of St. John's Wort in managing mild depression. In comparison to some pharmacological antidepressants, this herbal alternative is shown to be just as effective but with fewer side effects (Peterson & Nguyen, 2023). This could be quite appealing for those seeking a more natural approach to mental health without the burden of significant side effects. An analysis of clinical data suggests that St. John's Wort could offer relief from depressive symptoms, thanks largely to its ability to modulate certain neurotransmitters linked to mood regulation.

Historically, St. John's Wort has deep roots in herbal medicine. Ancient Greeks were among the first to utilize this vibrant flowering plant for its mood-enhancing properties. It was often used as part of rituals and medicinal practices aimed at elevating spirits and promoting emotional well-being (Henderson et al., 2002). The tradition continued across various cultures, maintaining its place as a go-to remedy for emotional healing over the centuries.

The efficacy of St. John's Wort is primarily attributed to two active compounds—hypericin and hyperforin. These constituents are believed to play a crucial role in affecting serotonin levels in the brain, similar to how many conventional antidepressants operate. By enhancing serotonin availability, these compounds may help stabilize mood and alleviate depressive symptoms. Importantly, hyperforin is recognized for its influence on multiple neurotransmitter systems beyond serotonin, potentially offering a broader spectrum of mood support.

While the therapeutic potential of St. John's Wort is promising, it is essential to be aware of safety considerations. Interactions with conventional antidepressants can present significant risks. For instance, combining St. John's Wort with selective serotonin reuptake inhibitors or other antidepressants can lead to serotonin syndrome, a condition characterized by excessive stimulation of the central nervous system that can be life-threatening if not addressed promptly. This underscores the importance of consulting healthcare professionals before beginning any regimen involving St. John's Wort, particularly for those already taking prescribed medications (Peterson & Nguyen, 2023).

Practical use and consideration guidelines are pivotal. Before incorporating St. John's Wort into your wellness routine, discuss your intentions with a healthcare provider who understands both herbal and traditional pharmaceutical treatments. They can provide personalized guidance based on your current health status and medication profile, ensuring that you harness the benefits of St. John's Wort safely and effectively. It's also advisable to source quality products from reputable manufacturers to ensure you receive a potent formulation of the herb.

## Bringing It All Together

Throughout this chapter, we've explored how ancient herbal practices are being revived and validated through modern scientific research. By contemplating the anti-inflammatory properties of turmeric, the immune-boosting power of Echinacea, and the mood-enhancing effects of St. John's Wort, we've seen a fascinating blend of old wisdom and new evidence. These herbs, with their roots in traditional medicine, offer accessible ways to enhance health naturally. It's intriguing to see how our ancestors' knowledge continues to find its place in today's world, proving that natural treatments can be both trusted and effective.

As we embrace these herbal remedies, it's important to stay informed about how they fit into our lives today. Whether you're looking to incorporate turmeric into your diet, experiment with Echinacea during flu season, or explore St. John's Wort for emotional well-being, the key is balance and understanding. Always consult with healthcare professionals to ensure these natural options complement your lifestyle safely. Remember, while nature offers incredible solutions, how we use them makes all the difference. So, as you consider using these age-old herbs, do so with an open mind and careful consideration.

# Chapter 10: The Future of Herbal Medicine

The future of herbal medicine is all about integrating ancient wisdom with modern healthcare practices. As we move forward, there's a growing interest in how these two approaches can work together to provide more comprehensive patient care. The rich history of using herbs for healing has long been overshadowed by conventional medicine, but now, people are beginning to see the value in combining both.

While traditional practitioners have relied on herbs for centuries, incorporating them into today's medical field opens up new possibilities for improving health outcomes. With the right balance, herbal medicine might play a significant role in offering holistic solutions that address not just symptoms but also the root causes of ailments. As we look ahead, this blend of old and new could be key to advancing healthcare.

In this chapter, we'll explore the exciting prospect of integrating herbal medicine within modern healthcare systems. We'll consider the collaborative practices between doctors and herbalists and the benefits of including herbal treatments in insurance coverage. You'll learn about the training opportunities available for healthcare providers to better understand the potential of herbal remedies. We'll also discuss the importance of policy development to ensure safe and effective use of these treatments.

By examining these aspects, we aim to highlight the impact and potential that herbal medicine holds for the future. Whether through teamwork among healthcare professionals or increased accessibility through insurance and education, this chapter uncovers how herbal medicine might reshape healthcare for the better.

## Herbal Medicine in Modern Healthcare Systems

In recent years, there has been a resurgence of interest in herbal remedies, driven by a growing desire for natural, holistic health solutions. As more people seek alternatives to conventional treatments, herbal medicine is making its way back into mainstream healthcare discussions. This renewed focus on plant-based healing offers exciting possibilities for the future, particularly when it comes to integrating traditional herbal practices with modern healthcare systems.

### Collaboration Between Traditional and Modern Medicine

The future of healthcare increasingly points toward collaboration between healthcare professionals and herbalists. By blending the knowledge of both traditional herbal medicine and conventional medicine, we can create more holistic and effective treatment plans. This integration allows for a broader approach, addressing not just symptoms but the root causes of health issues. Countries such as China and India, where herbal medicine and modern treatments have coexisted for centuries, offer valuable examples of how this can be done effectively. This collaborative model fosters a more inclusive and patient-centered approach to health (Zhang et al., 2011).

## Expanding Access Through Insurance Coverage

As the interest in herbal medicine grows, one of the major barriers to its widespread adoption is the lack of insurance coverage for herbal treatments. Many patients who wish to explore herbal remedies are left to pay out-of-pocket, limiting access, particularly for those who could benefit the most.

The future of healthcare would benefit greatly from expanding insurance policies to cover herbal treatments, reflecting the increasing demand for integrative health options. By including herbal medicine in insurance plans, patients gain more freedom in their healthcare choices, empowering them to pursue holistic treatment methods.

Pilot programs by insurance companies could be a first step in gathering data on patient satisfaction and the cost-effectiveness of these treatments, ultimately guiding policy changes (*Traditional, Complementary and Integrative Medicine*, n.d.).

## Training Healthcare Providers for the Future

For the resurgence of herbal medicine to truly integrate into modern healthcare, healthcare providers must be educated about the benefits and uses of herbs. As demand for natural remedies increases, it becomes crucial that doctors have the necessary knowledge to advise patients about herbal treatments. Some medical institutions, such as those in Australia and the United States, have already begun to offer courses on complementary and alternative medicine, acknowledging the growing interest in these practices. The future of healthcare lies in providing healthcare professionals with the foundational knowledge they need to engage in informed discussions with patients and recommend holistic treatments when appropriate (Zhang et al., 2011).

## Establishing Clear Regulatory Guidelines

Establishing clear regulatory policies is essential to ensure the safe and effective use of herbal remedies. Strong regulations can ensure that herbal products meet high-quality standards, maintain safety, and provide consistent results. Regulatory bodies like the WHO have emphasized the need for standards and guidelines to ensure the effectiveness and safety of herbal treatments. Moving forward, governments and healthcare organizations must continue to push for research funding and policy development that supports the safe integration of herbal medicine into clinical practice (*Traditional, Complementary and Integrative Medicine*, n.d.).

## Impact of Technology on Herbal Medicine Research

In recent years, technology has been rapidly transforming various fields, and herbal medicine is no exception. The integration of technological advancements offers exciting prospects for improving the study and application of herbal remedies. By leveraging data analysis, research innovations, online platforms, and telemedicine, we can make herbal medicine more effective, accessible, and credible than ever before.

First, let's talk about data analysis techniques. For a long time, herbal medicine relied heavily on traditional knowledge passed down through generations. While this approach has its merits, it often lacks the rigorous scientific backing that contemporary data analysis can provide.

With big data tools, researchers can now sift through vast amounts of information to identify patterns and trends in the efficacy of different herbs. This not only enhances the credibility of herbal studies but also helps in pinpointing which compounds are most beneficial.

Imagine being able to cross-reference thousands of studies and patient records to determine how a specific herb affects blood pressure or mental health. Such evidence-based practices elevate herbal medicine from folklore to a scientifically validated field (Junaid et al., 2022).

Next, research innovations have taken center stage in uncovering the mysteries of herbs. For example, advances in molecular biology allow scientists to isolate and identify the active compounds within plants. This means we can now understand precisely what makes chamomile calming or ginger digestive.

By analyzing these compounds, researchers can develop more effective formulations and dosages tailored to specific health conditions. Moreover, these innovations open up possibilities for synthesizing concentrated forms of herbal remedies. This could lead to more potent treatments with fewer side effects (Senbekov et al., 2020).

Moving onto the digital world, online platforms have revolutionized how we access information. In the past, learning about herbal medicine might have meant flipping through dusty books or attending local workshops. Today, however, digital resources abound, making herbal knowledge available at our fingertips.

Websites, apps, and online courses offer comprehensive guides on everything from identifying herbs to preparing them for use. This democratization of knowledge empowers individuals to educate themselves about natural remedies, fostering a more informed public. Furthermore, online reviews and forums create spaces for users to share their experiences and findings, enriching the collective understanding of herbal medicine.

Telemedicine is another game-changer in expanding access to herbal consultations. Traditional healthcare often requires patients to physically visit clinics, which can be inconvenient or even impossible for those living in remote areas.

Telehealth services bridge this gap by allowing patients to consult with herbalists virtually. This not only broadens access but also enables people to explore alternative treatments they might not find locally. Through video calls and chat services, patients can discuss their symptoms and receive personalized recommendations from experts, all without leaving their homes. This shift toward virtual consultations aligns with a growing desire for more holistic and patient-centered healthcare models.

However, integrating technology into herbal medicine does come without challenges. Ensuring data privacy and security is paramount, particularly when dealing with sensitive health information. Additionally, while online resources provide convenient access, they must be curated and validated to prevent the spread of misinformation. Regulatory bodies play a crucial role here, establishing guidelines to ensure the safety and quality of digital health products and services.

Moreover, technology should complement rather than replace the traditional aspects of herbal medicine. Cultural wisdom and empirical experiences still hold invaluable insights that technology cannot replicate. The goal is to blend these two worlds, enhancing what's tried and true with what's cutting edge.

Returning to telemedicine, it's essential to establish clear guidelines to optimize its benefits. Reliable internet connections, user-friendly interfaces, and training for both practitioners and patients on digital tools can significantly enhance the experience. These steps ensure that individuals, regardless of technological skill, can effectively engage with herbal consultants online, empowering them to take charge of their health.

## Keeping Ancient Herbal Knowledge Alive

Preserving and passing on the ancient knowledge of herbal medicine to future generations is crucial in maintaining the historical and cultural richness of these practices. By focusing on specific strategies, we can ensure that this valuable knowledge doesn't get lost over time.

First off, documentation and preservation play a pivotal role in safeguarding traditional uses of herbs. This isn't just about jotting down recipes or remedies; it's about capturing the essence of an entire way of life that has been passed through generations.

For example, consider ancient healing texts like the Ebers Papyrus or the Ayurvedic Samhitas, which provide invaluable insights into past civilizations' medical practices (Elendu, 2024). In the same vein, modern efforts could involve compiling written records, oral histories, and even video documentaries that encapsulate traditional herbal practices.

Documentation serves as a bridge, connecting the old with the new. It provides a robust foundation for future research and applications. Researchers today often rely on such documentation to identify the medicinal properties of herbs, a process akin to detective work, piecing together cultural wisdom with scientific inquiry. This collaboration not only preserves history but also enhances our understanding of herbal efficacy and potential integration into contemporary medicine.

Another effective approach to preserving ancient herbal knowledge is through community workshops. These workshops aren't merely educational sessions; they are dynamic spaces where knowledge is shared, skills are honed, and communities are strengthened.

Picture a room bustling with enthusiasts, both young and old, gathered around tables laden with fresh herbs, learning the nuances of traditional healing methods. Here, theory meets practice, turning abstract knowledge into tangible skills. Workshops can provide guidelines on how to cultivate, harvest, and use various herbs safely and effectively, making them accessible to everyone interested in herbalism.

Such interactive settings are excellent for fostering a sense of belonging and continuity within the community of herbal practitioners. They become safe havens where questions can be asked freely, and experiences are shared openly. This environment not only facilitates hands-on learning but also ignites passion and curiosity in novice herbalists, ensuring continued interest and development in the field.

Mentorship programs further amplify the transmission of herbal expertise. Experienced herbalists stepping into mentorship roles can guide novices through the intricate landscape of herbal medicine, much like a master-apprentice relationship. This personal connection allows for deeper learning and encourages innovation within the traditional framework. Novices benefit immensely from the wealth of experience that seasoned herbalists bring, making the learning process not just informative but transformative.

Mentorship goes beyond structured learning; it builds relationships and networks that are essential for any field's growth. As mentees learn directly from experienced professionals, they gain unique insights and practical skills that textbooks alone cannot provide. Moreover, these programs foster innovation by encouraging new ideas to flourish under the guidance of established experts, blending time-tested techniques with contemporary perspectives.

In today's digital age, online educational courses have become a powerful tool to broaden the reach of herbal education globally. These courses offer flexibility and accessibility, allowing anyone with an internet connection to delve into the world of herbal medicine. Whether it's a short course on identifying local flora or an in-depth dive into advanced herbal pharmacology, online platforms make quality herbal education available to a diverse audience.

Online courses provide legitimacy to herbal studies by offering structured learning paths and certified qualifications. They help break down geographical barriers, enabling a cross-cultural exchange of knowledge and bringing a global perspective to traditional practices. For instance, someone in America can learn about Ayurveda through Indian experts, or a student in Europe might study Amazonian herbal traditions taught by South American healers. This interconnectedness enriches the learning experience and strengthens global appreciation for herbal medicine.

Moreover, these courses often incorporate multimedia resources, live demonstrations, and interactive forums, creating an engaging learning atmosphere. They can complement traditional learning methods, giving aspiring herbalists a comprehensive education that's both flexible and comprehensive. By integrating modern technology with ancient wisdom, online courses empower more individuals to explore and contribute to the field of herbal medicine.

## Bringing It All Together

Now that we've looked at the evolving role of herbal medicine in future healthcare, it's clearer than ever that integrating herbal medicine with modern medical practices is not just possible but promising. By encouraging collaboration between doctors and herbalists, we can create well-rounded treatment plans that truly cater to individual patient needs.

The idea is not to replace conventional medicine but to complement it, offering patients a wider range of safe and effective options. Likewise, expanding insurance coverage for herbal treatments can make these alternatives more accessible, allowing people from all walks of life to explore them without financial strain.

Education and policy development are key areas that need attention if we're to fully integrate herbal medicine into mainstream healthcare. Training healthcare providers in herbal knowledge ensures they can discuss these options confidently with patients, while careful regulation ensures safety and efficacy across the board.

Furthermore, leveraging technology offers exciting opportunities to refine and expand our understanding of herbal treatments, making high-quality information widely available. As traditional wisdom meets cutting-edge innovation, we find ourselves on the brink of a healthcare model that's holistic, inclusive, and forward-thinking.

# Conclusion

As our exploration into herbal health comes to a close, we celebrate the fusion of ancient wisdom and modern innovation, offering a holistic path to wellness. Nature's enduring remedies, like chamomile and rosemary blends, remind us of the power within each herb to nurture and heal. Embracing these traditions alongside today's advancements invites you to not just add remedies to your toolkit but also build a mindset of lifelong learning.

Your journey into herbal health will involve cultivating a deeper, more personalized connection with your well-being, both physically and spiritually.

Let the wisdom of the past and the promise of the future guide you on this path of continuous discovery!

# Quick Reference Guide

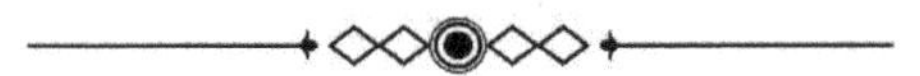

The following table provides a comprehensive list of herbal recipes and remedies, organized by their intended use. Whether you're seeking relief from common ailments, looking to boost your immune system, or simply wanting to incorporate natural remedies into your routine, these recipes offer practical, time-tested solutions derived from nature's pharmacy. Each remedy includes a brief description of its use to help you easily find what you need.

| Name | Category (Use) | Description | Page No. |
|---|---|---|---|
| **Honey Throat Soother** | Sore Throat Relief | A warm honey-based drink to soothe irritation. | 46 |
| **Peppermint Digestive Tea** | Digestive Aid | An herbal tea that eases stomach cramps and digestion. | 47 |

| **Aloe Vera Skin Soother** | Skin Irritations and Burns | A cooling gel to relieve skin irritation and burns. | 48 |
|---|---|---|---|
| **Ginger Tea** | Nausea and Digestion | A warming tea to ease nausea and support digestion. | 48 |
| **Garlic-Infused Oil** | Immune and Antimicrobia l Support | An oil used for cooking or as a topical antimicrobial. | 49 |
| **Turmeric Golden Milk** | Anti-Inflammator y | A warm, spiced drink with turmeric for reducing inflammation. | 49 |
| **Chamomile Tea** | Relaxation and Digestion | A calming tea for stress relief and digestion. | 50 |
| **Tea Tree Oil Treatment** | Skin Blemishes and Minor Cuts | A topical antiseptic for acne and wounds. | 51 |

| | | | |
|---|---|---|---|
| **Cinnamon Water** | Blood Sugar Regulation | A drink that helps regulate blood sugar and soothes the throat. | 51 |
| **Lemon Garlic Tonic** | Immune Booster | A blend of lemon, garlic, and honey for immunity. | 52 |
| **Hibiscus Tea** | Heart Health and Blood Pressure | A vibrant tea for lowering blood pressure and heart support. | 52 |
| **Chamomile Herbal Bath** | Stress Relief and Skin Soother | A relaxing bath soak for calming effects. | 53 |
| **Basil Water** | Hydration and Digestion | A refreshing drink for hydration and digestive support. | 53 |
| **Willow Bark Tea** | Pain Relief and Anti- | A natural tea for pain relief. | 20 |

| | | | |
|---|---|---|---|
| | Inflammatory | | |
| **Willow Bark Tincture** | Pain Relief | A concentrated herbal extract for pain management. | 21 |
| **Garlic and Honey Remedy** | Immune and Antiviral Support | A mix of crushed garlic and honey for boosting immunity. | 23 |
| **Mint and Cucumber Cooler** | Hydration and Headache Relief | A cooling drink for hydration and headache relief. | 54 |
| **Lemon Balm Tea** | Stress and Anxiety Relief | A tea that promotes relaxation and eases anxiety. | 62 |
| **Valerian Root Tea** | Sleep and Anxiety Aid | A tea to promote restful sleep and calm the | 63 |

| | | | |
|---|---|---|---|
| | | nervous system. | |
| **Sage Smudging Ritual** | Energy Cleansing | A sage bundle for purification and spiritual cleansing. | 80 |
| **Calendula Ointment** | Wound Healing | An antiseptic ointment for minor cuts and scrapes. | 33 |
| **Arnica Compress** | Bruising and Swelling Relief | A compress to reduce bruising and swelling. | 33 |
| **Yarrow Tea** | Fever Reduction | A tea to help induce sweating and reduce fever. | 34 |
| **Sage Infusion** | Antiseptic and Fever Reduction | A sage-based infusion for fighting infections. | 34 |
| **Ginseng Tea** | Vitality and Focus | A revitalizing tea for | 23 |

| | | | |
|---|---|---|---|
| | | boosting energy and concentration. | |
| **Ginseng Tincture** | Energy and Immune Support | A concentrated herbal extract to enhance resilience. | 24 |

# FREE GIFT

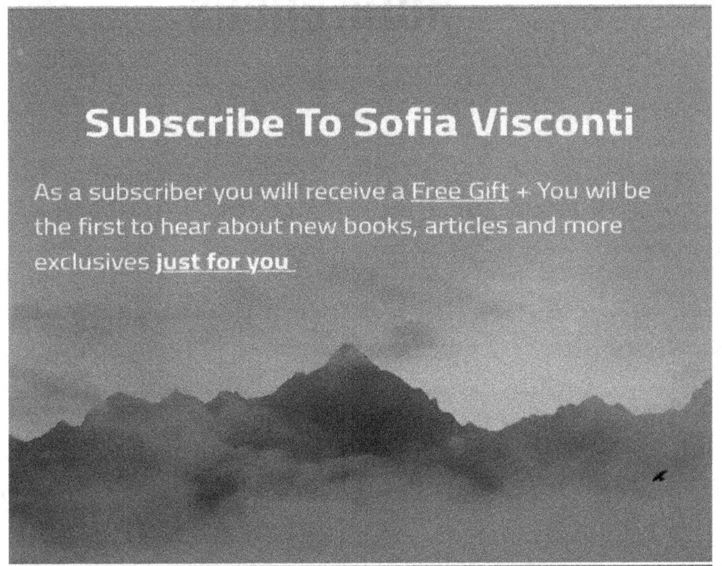


CLICK HERE

Or Visit Below:

https://www.subscribepage.com/svmyth

Simply scan the QR code to join.

# References

*American ginseng.* (n.d.). Mount Sinai. https://www.mountsinai.org/health-library/herb/american-ginseng

*Ancient Greek medicine.* (2008). National Library of Medicine. https://www.nlm.nih.gov/hmd/topics/greek-medicine/index.html

Ankri, S., & Mirelman, D. (1999). Antimicrobial properties of allicin from garlic. *Microbes and Infection, 1*(2), 125–129. https://doi.org/10.1016/s1286-4579(99)80003-3

Axe, J. (2022, December 3). *10 lavender oil benefits for major diseases & minor ailments.* Dr. Axe. https://draxe.com/essential-oils/lavender-oil-benefits/

Baek, J. H., Nierenberg, A. A., & Kinrys, G. (2014). Clinical applications of herbal medicines for anxiety and insomnia; targeting patients with bipolar disorder. *Australian & New Zealand Journal of Psychiatry, 48*(8), 705–715. https://doi.org/10.1177/0004867414539198

Bhatwalkar, S. B., Mondal, R., Krishna, S. B. N., Adam, J. K., Govender, P., & Anupam, R. (2021). Antibacterial properties of organosulfur compounds of garlic (Allium sativum). *Frontiers in Microbiology, 12*(613077). https://doi.org/10.3389/fmicb.2021.613077

Bharathi, G., Saravan, K., & Bharathi, A. (2025, January 11). *The history and traditions of herbal medicine: An overview.* Research Gate. https://www.researchgate.net/publication/388185872_The_History_and_Traditions_of_Herbal_Medicine_An_Overview

*Blue cohosh: Overview, uses, side effects, and more.* (n.d.). WebMD. https://www.webmd.com/vitamins/ai/ingredientmono-987/blue-cohosh

Boeck, B. (2020, October 28). *Investigating the healing arts of Ancient Mesopotamia.* Research Outreach. https://researchoutreach.org/articles/investigating-healing-arts-ancient-mesopotamia/

CARE medical team. (2023, August 8). *Benefits of fenugreek seeds.* Care Hospitals. https://www.carehospitals.com/blog-detail/benefits-of-fenugreek-seed/

Carr, M. (2014, October 13). *Mummies and the usefulness of death.* Science History Institute. https://www.sciencehistory.org/stories/magazine/mummies-and-the-usefulness-of-death/

Chumpitazi, B. P., Kearns, G. L., & Shulman, R. J. (2018). Review article: the physiological effects and safety of peppermint oil and its efficacy in irritable bowel syndrome and other functional disorders. *Alimentary Pharmacology & Therapeutics*, *47*(6), 738–752. https://doi.org/10.1111/apt.14519

Daily, J. W., Yang, M., & Park, S. (2016). Efficacy of turmeric extracts and curcumin for alleviating the symptoms of joint arthritis: A systematic review and meta-analysis of randomized clinical trials. *Journal of Medicinal Food*, *19*(8), 717–729. https://doi.org/10.1089/jmf.2016.3705

Dudley, N., Higgins-Zogib, L., & Mansourian, S. (2009). The links between protected areas, faiths, and sacred natural sites. *Conservation Biology*, *23*(3), 568–577. https://doi.org/10.1111/j.1523-1739.2009.01201.x

*Echinacea.* (2024a). Mount Sinai. https://www.mountsinai.org/health-library/herb/echinacea

*Echinacea.* (2024b, October). National Library of Medicine. https://www.nccih.nih.gov/health/echinacea

Elendu, C. (2024). The evolution of ancient healing practices: From shamanism to Hippocratic medicine: A review. *Medicine*, *103*(28), e39005. https://doi.org/10.1097/MD.0000000000039005

Eteraf-Oskouei, T., & Najafi, M. (2012). Traditional and modern uses of natural honey in human diseases: A review. *Iranian Journal of Basic Medical Sciences*, *16*(6), 731. https://pmc.ncbi.nlm.nih.gov/articles/PMC3758027/

*Four sacred medicines.* (n.d.). Aihschgo. https://aihschgo.org/four-sacred-medicines/

*A guide to traditional herbalism across cultures.* (2024, April 15). Gaia Herbs. https://www.gaiaherbs.com/blogs/seeds-of-knowledge/herbalism-folk-medicine?srsltid=AfmBOooCTfT43k2LUTIXT1uE_nva6vI8RPSHvplRHnGgLTc63FzzvHBX

Gupta, S., Srivastava, J. K., & Shankar, E. (2010). Chamomile: A herbal medicine of the past with a bright future. *Molecular Medicine Reports*, *3*(6). https://doi.org/10.3892/mmr.2010.377

Hassen, G., Belete, G., Carrera, K. G., Iriowen, R. O., Araya, H., Alemu, T., Solomon, N., Bam, D. S., Nicola, S. M., Araya, M. E., Debele, T., Zouetr, M., & Jain, N. (2022). Clinical implications of herbal supplements in conventional medical practice: A US perspective. *Cureus*, *14*(7). https://doi.org/10.7759/cureus.26893

Hekmatpou, D., Mehrabi, F., Rahzani, K., & Aminiyan, A. (2017). The effect of aloe vera clinical trials on prevention and healing of skin wound: A systematic review. *Iranian Journal of Medical Sciences*, *44*(1), 1. https://pmc.ncbi.nlm.nih.gov/articles/PMC6330525/

Henderson, L., Yue, Q. Y., Bergquist, C., Gerden, B., & Arlett, P. (2002). St John's wort (Hypericum perforatum): Drug interactions and clinical outcomes. *British Journal of Clinical Pharmacology*, *54*(4), 349–356. https://doi.org/10.1046/j.1365-2125.2002.01683.x

*Hyssop (Niu Xi Cao)*. (2023, December 5). White Rabbit Institute of Healing. https://www.whiterabbitinstituteofhealing.com/herbs/hyssop/

Icahn School of Medicine at Mount Sinai. (n.d.). *Willow bark information.* Mount Sinai Health System. https://www.mountsinai.org/health-library/herb/willow-bark

Jahromi, B., Pirvulescu, I., Candido, K. D., & Knezevic, N. N. (2021). Herbal medicine for pain management: Efficacy and drug interactions. *Pharmaceutics*, *13*(2), 251. https://doi.org/10.3390/pharmaceutics13020251

Jasiński, J. (n.d.). *Herbs used in ancient Rome.* Imperium Romanum. https://imperiumromanum.pl/en/roman-society/eating-habits-of-romans/herbs-used-in-ancient-rome/

Junaid, S. B., Imam, A. A., Balogun, A. O., De Silva, L. C., Surakat, Y. A., Kumar, G., Abdulkarim, M., Shuaibu, A. N., Garba, A., Sahalu, Y., Mohammed, A., Mohammed, T. Y., Abdulkadir, B. A., Abba, A. A., Kakumi, N. A. I., & Mahamad, S. (2022). Recent advancements in emerging technologies for healthcare management systems: A survey. *Healthcare*, *10*(10), 1–45. https://doi.org/10.3390/healthcare10101940

Kenda, M., Kočevar Glavač, N., Nagy, M., & Sollner Dolenc, M. (2022). Medicinal plants used for anxiety, depression, or stress treatment: An update. *Molecules*, *27*(18), 6021. https://doi.org/10.3390/molecules27186021

Kou, H., Huang, L., Jin, M., He, Q., Zhang, R., & Ma, J. (2023). Effect of curcumin on rheumatoid arthritis: a systematic review and meta-analysis. *Frontiers in*

*Immunology*, *14*. https://doi.org/10.3389/fimmu.2023.1121655

Larkin, B. (2023). *A-Z guide for burning sage: History, benefits, & how-to smudge!* Tiny Rituals. https://tinyrituals.co/blogs/tiny-rituals/burning-sage?srsltid=AfmBOoonno_OEgI4y10ao47BGDBx09krqG153M84wsbxTjlJ998Teq-k

Lin, C.-R., Huang, S., Che, W., Lee, C., Hung, S.-W., Ting, Y. M., & Hung, Y. (2023). Willow bark (Salix spp.) used for pain relief in arthritis: A meta-analysis of randomized controlled trials. *Life*, *13*(10), 2058–2058. https://doi.org/10.3390/life13102058

Mandal, M. D., & Mandal, S. (2011). Honey: Its medicinal property and antibacterial activity. *Asian Pacific Journal of Tropical Biomedicine*, *1*(2), 154–160. https://doi.org/10.1016/s2221-1691(11)60016-6

McFarlin, B. L., Gibson, M. H., O'Rear, J., & Harman, P. (1999). A national survey of herbal preparation use by nurse-midwives for labor stimulation. Review of the literature and recommendations for practice. *Journal of Nurse-Midwifery*, *44*(3), 205–216. https://doi.org/10.1016/s0091-2182(99)00037-3

*The mentorship program*. (2025, January 8). Ann Cecil-Sterman. https://anncecilsterman.com/mp25/

Metwaly, A. M., Ghoneim, M. M., Eissa, Ibrahim. H., Elsehemy, I. A., Mostafa, A. E., Hegazy, M. M., Afifi, W. M., & Dou, D. (2021). Traditional Ancient Egyptian medicine: A review. *Saudi Journal of Biological Sciences, 28*(10). https://doi.org/10.1016/j.sjbs.2021.06.044

Norman, J. (2014, December 27). *Knowledge as power: King Ashurbanipal forms the earliest systematically collected library as distinct from an archive.* History of Information. https://www.historyofinformation.com/detail.php?id=8

Nguyen, M. (2024, December 16). *The spiritual power of sage: Ancient practices for cleansing and renewal.* Sacred Plant Co. https://sacredplantco.com/blogs/natures-pharmacy-exploring-the-historical-uses-and-health-benefits-of-medicinal-herbs/the-spiritual-power-of-sage-ancient-practices-for-cleansing-and-renewal?srsltid=AfmBOorj7ylb6IQP4COxqrh5x7BmawJOdVMR6wPtvZR88Fy8H7u_8mL4

*Our ingredients.* (2022, March 30). Herbaceous Skincare. https://www.herbaceousskincare.com/ingredients/

Patterson, R. (2018, May 22). *Devas/plant spirits.* Witches and Pagans. https://witchesandpagans.com/pagan-paths-blogs/hedge-witch/devas-plant-spirits.html

*Peppermint oil.* (2020, October). National Library of Medicine. https://www.nccih.nih.gov/health/peppermint-oil

Peterson, B., & Nguyen, H. (2023, May 16). *St. John's Wort.* National Library of Medicine; StatPearls Publishing. https://www.ncbi.nlm.nih.gov/books/NBK557465/

Petran, M., Dragos, D., & Gilca, M. (2020). Historical ethnobotanical review of medicinal plants used to treat children diseases in Romania (1860s–1970s). *Journal of Ethnobiology and Ethnomedicine*, *16*(1). https://doi.org/10.1186/s13002-020-00364-6

Sah, A., Naseef, P. P., Kuruniyan, M. S., Jain, G. K., Zakir, F., & Aggarwal, G. (2022). A comprehensive study of therapeutic applications of chamomile. *Pharmaceuticals*, *15*(10), 1284. https://doi.org/10.3390/ph15101284

Senbekov, M., Saliev, T., Bukeyeva, Z., Almabayeva, A., Zhanaliyeva, M., Aitenova, N., Toishibekov, Y., & Fakhradiyev, I. (2020). The recent progress and applications of digital technologies in healthcare: a review. *International Journal of Telemedicine and Applications*, *2020*(1), 1–18.

Shaban, D., & Cameron, K. (2025, January 30). *Health benefits of fenugreek*. WebMD. https://www.webmd.com/diet/health-benefits-of-fenugreek

Socha, M. W., Flis, W., Wartęga, M., Szambelan, M., Pietrus, M., & Kazdepka-Ziemińska, A. (2023). Raspberry leaves and extracts—Molecular mechanism of action and its effectiveness on human cervical ripening and the induction of labor. *Nutrients*, *15*(14), 3206. https://doi.org/10.3390/nu15143206

*The soothing benefits of a lavender candle.* (2024, July 24). Ahuru Candles. https://www.ahurucandles.co.nz/blogs/guide/lavender-candle?srsltid=AfmBOoqVQy-XYd6AVopJuoNCgTN4_DfvvHvBmIyBzwP2VYHUv_DbGZY

Surjushe, A., Vasani, R., & Saple, D. (2008). Aloe vera: A short review. *Indian Journal of Dermatology, 53*(4), 163. https://doi.org/10.4103/0019-5154.44785

Torrens, K. (2022, December 16). *Top 9 health benefits of raspberry leaf tea.* Good Food. https://www.bbcgoodfood.com/health/nutrition/top-9-health-benefits-of-raspberry-leaf-tea

Totelin, L. (2014). When foods become remedies in ancient Greece: The curious case of garlic and other substances. *Journal of Ethnopharmacology, 167*, 30–37. https://doi.org/10.1016/j.jep.2014.08.018

*Traditional, complementary and integrative medicine.* (n.d.). World Health Organization. https://www.who.int/teams/integrated-health-services/traditional-complementary-and-integrative-medicine

*Traditional teaching.* (n.d.). Mushkiki. https://mushkiki.com/programs-services/the-four-sacred-medicines/

Wee, J. J., Mee Park, K., & Chung, A.-S. (2011). *Biological activities of ginseng and its application to human health* (I. F. F. Benzie & S. Wachtel-Galor, Eds.). National Library of Medicine; CRC Press/Taylor & Francis. https://www.ncbi.nlm.nih.gov/books/NBK92776/

*Willow bark*. (n.d.). Mount Sinai. https://www.mountsinai.org/health-library/herb/willow-bark

*Willow is a valuable medicine for rheumatic conditions*. (2025, February 17). Herbal Reality. https://www.herbalreality.com/herb/white-willow/

Yogi, W., Tsukada, M., Sato, Y., Izuno, T., Inoue, T., Tsunokawa, Y., Okumo, T., Hisamitsu, T., & Sunagawa, M. (2021). Influences of lavender essential oil inhalation on stress responses during short-duration sleep cycles: A pilot study. *Healthcare*, *9*(7), 909. https://doi.org/10.3390/healthcare9070909

Zhang, A.L., Changli Xue, C., & Fong, H. H. S. (2011). *Integration of herbal medicine into evidence-based clinical practice*. National Library of Medicine; CRC Press/Taylor & Francis. https://www.ncbi.nlm.nih.gov/books/NBK92760/

www.ingramcontent.com/pod-product-compliance
Lightning Source LLC
Chambersburg PA
CBHW050214270326
41914CB00003BA/411
* 9 7 8 1 0 8 8 1 3 4 2 5 2 *